Tu Youyou — China's First Female Nobel Prize Winner

Liu Liping

Published by
ACA Publishing Ltd.
University House
11-13 Lower Grosvenor Place
London SW1W 0EX, UK
Tel: +44 (0)20 7834 7676
Fax: +44 (0)20 7973 0076
E-mail: info@alaincharlesasia.com
Web: www.alaincharlesasia.com
Beijing Office
Tel: +86(0)10 8472 1250
Fax: +86(0)10 5885 0639

Authors: Liu Liping
Editor: David
Translator: Zhang Mingfang
Cover art: Daniel Li

Published by ACA Publishing Ltd in association
with the People's Publishing House

ISBN 978-1-910760-18-5

A catalogue record for *Tu Youyou — China's First Female Nobel Prize Winner*
is available from the National Bibliographic Service of the British Library.

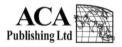

Contents

Foreword

At 11.30am local time on October 5, 2015, the hall of the Karovinska Institutet, a medical university in the Swedish capital of Stockholm, was crowded with journalists from all over the world. Facing a large audience, Worben Lindale, executive secretary of the Nobel Committee for Physiology or Medicine, stepped on the dais with three judges.

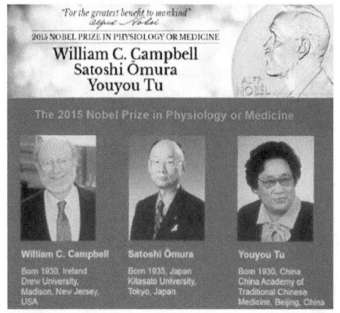

This photo was released on the official website of the Nobel prize on October 5, 2015. From left to right: William C. Campbell, the Irish scientist; Satoshi Ōmura, the Japanese scientist, and Tu Youyou, the Chinese pharmacologist

A smiling Worben Lindale declared in both Swedish and English that the 2015 Nobel prize in physiology or medicine was awarded to the Chinese pharmacologist Tu Youyou and another two scientists, William C. Campbell and Satoshi Ōmura, in recognition of their achievements in research into the treatment of parasitic diseases. The value of the award was 8m Swedish krona (around US$920,000). Tu Youyou received half of the award, with the other two scientists sharing the remainder.

While Lindale was announcing the news, the photos and profiles of the three prize-winners appeared on a screen behind him. In her photo, a bespectacled Tu Youyou was looking straight ahead with a slight smile on her face. Underneath was a brief introduction: "Born 1930, China – the China Academy of Chinese Medical Sciences, Beijing, China."

At that time it was 5.30pm in Beijing, on October 5, 2015. Tu Youyou was unaware that she had suddenly become a globally sought-after interviewee. She was taking a bath when her husband saw the news on television in their living room and told her immediately: "You have won the award."

At first, Tu Youyou gave the news little thought since she believed it concerned a less prestigious award, the Warren Alpert Foundation prize. Yet in no time, she received a flurry of congratulation letters and flowers. Journalists competed to secure an interview with her. She was unaccustomed to the sudden popularity brought about by her status as a Nobel prize winner. Everyone was extremely excited by the news. In winning this prestigious award, Tu Youyou set several new records: the first Chinese woman to win this Nobel prize; the highest international award obtained in China's medical history; and the highest award granted to achievements in traditional Chinese medicine.

At 1pm Beijing time on October 6, 2015, Lindale phoned Tu to officially congratulate her on winning the prize and sincerely invited her to attend the award ceremony in December 2015 in Sweden. In her 80s, Tu Youyou kept calm as usual. She told Lindale: "This is not only my personal honor, but also recognition from the international community for all Chinese scientific researchers."

The Nobel prize is not only a great honor, but also an affirmation of Tu Youyou's several decades of quiet and patient labor.

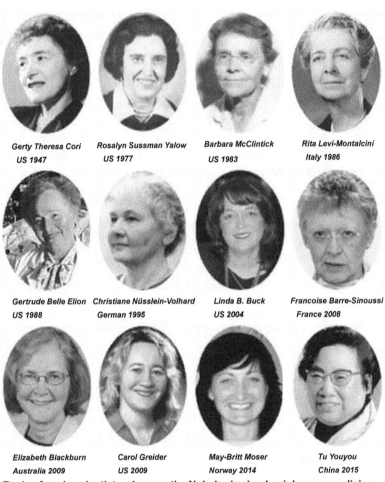

Gerty Theresa Cori
US 1947

Rosalyn Sussman Yalow
US 1977

Barbara McClintick
US 1983

Rita Levi-Montalcini
Italy 1986

Gertrude Belle Elion
US 1988

Christiane Nüsslein-Volhard
German 1995

Linda B. Buck
US 2004

Francoise Barre-Sinoussi
France 2008

Elizabeth Blackburn
Australia 2009

Carol Greider
US 2009

May-Britt Moser
Norway 2014

Tu Youyou
China 2015

Twelve female scientists who won the Nobel prize in physiology or medicine

A peaceful heart, indifference to fame and wealth, and courage in the pursuit of truth are all perhaps essential traits of great scientists. Numerous and repeated scientific research and experiments require patience, so it's impossible to conquer the fear and confusion of failure, make breakthroughs and obtain remarkable achievements without extraordinary perseverance and high ideals.

It may be true that favorable conditions are crucial in scientific innovation; however, extraordinary insight, broad vision and strong belief play the most significant roles. In order to ensure the safety of her patients, Tu Youyou actually took the medicines herself to test their effects. She went to an area in Hainan province with a malaria risk to obtain first-hand clinical information. She administered medicines to patients in the scorching sun. This dedication originates from her innermost love and benevolence, which are the power source of 'persistence in the discovery of artemisinin'.

Eighty-six years ago, Tu Youyou's father referred to *The Book of Songs* when naming his daughter. He probably didn't foresee that her future career would be closely associated with the magical traditional herbal medicine of sweet wormwood (Artemisia annua), and nor could he envisage that his daughter would save countless lives by this traditional herbal medicine.

As the first Chinese female scientist to win the Nobel prize, what were her formative experiences and the major events in her life? This book charts the extraordinary life of this great scientist and acknowledges her inspirational work.

Chapter 1

The Budding Talent of Tu Youyou

Ningbo City and the Yao Residence in the 1930s

Unfold a map of China, and you will see that Ningbo is a port city.
The history of Ningbo dates back 7,000 years to the Hemudu
culture. In the Xia dynasty, Ningbo was called Yin; in the Tang dynasty,
it was known as Mingzhou. Ningbo became China's largest port city
thanks to its geographical advantages and frequent trade with other
countries, including ancient Japan and Goryeo (a dynasty in Korean
history). The further development of foreign trade made it the starting
point of the Maritime Silk Road. At the beginning of the Yuan dynasty
in 1271, Ningbo was a distribution center for goods transported
from both south and north China, and it was one of the nation's most
important ports. In the Qing dynasty, a well-known school specializing
in the study of the history of eastern Zhejiang province was established
in Ningbo, which helped to enhance exchanges between the city and
western countries. In 1844, two years after the first Opium War, Ningbo
was reopened to western countries, which damaged the local economy.
Just at that time, the Ningbo business community adopted modern
practices and turned to the emerging Shanghai as their major market,
greatly influencing Shanghai's urbanization and civilization. During the
period of the Republic of China, Ningbo's economy fluctuated due to
war. Between January and February 1927, the National Revolutionary
Army defeated soldiers headed by the warlord Sun Chuanfang and then
went on to occupy Ningbo. It was not until the 1930s that conflict and
turmoil eased in Ningbo.

Tu Youyou was born in Ningbo during these turbulent times.

At dawn on December 30, 1930, a baby uttered its first cry in the Tu family home at 508 Kaiming Road, Ningbo. With three boys in the household already, this baby was a long-cherished 'princess'.

Her crying resembled the 'yoyo' sound of a deer.

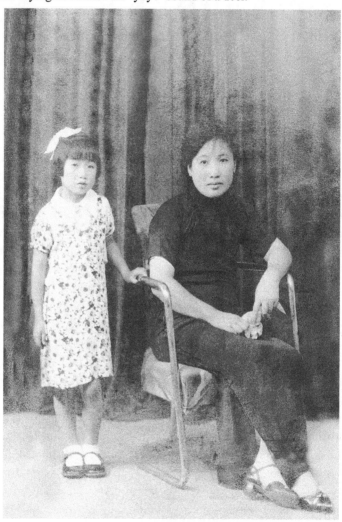

The earliest surviving photo of Tu Youyou, pictured here with her mother

Showered with happiness at the birth of Tu Youyou, her father Tu Liangui recited subconsciously this famous line from *The Book of Songs*: "Yo, yo, cries a herd of deer that eat wormwood in the wilderness."

In accordance with the Chinese tradition of naming girls from lines in *The Book of Songs* and boys from *The Book of Chu*, Tu Liangui gave his daughter the name Youyou. Therefore the sound 'yoyo' would always be present in the father's heart, reflecting his love, expectations and joy for his daughter.

After reciting the line "Yo, yo, cries a herd of deer that eat wormwood in the wilderness", her father came up with: "Being fresh and green, the wormwood appreciates the light of spring", making the lines more meaningful and perfect. These poetic lines would often feature in Tu Youyou's childhood.

The lines "Being fresh and green, the wormwood appreciates the light of spring" could have planted the wormwood seed in his daughter's destiny.

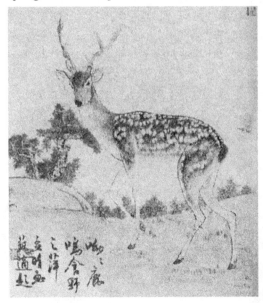

The traditional Chinese painting Deer's Call by Meng Qing

Tu Youyou's childhood years were spent in Kaiming Road, situated in the Lotus Bridge Mansion region in central Ningbo. Living here, she immersed herself in the most refined cultural district south of the Yangtze river.

This region was blessed with a favorable geographical location and rich natural resources that radiated in all directions. Bizarre folk acrobatics took place here, such as performances involving tall flag poles and carts pulled by ropes; native traditional arts such as shadow plays and puppet shows that made people dizzy with wonder. Wandering in the commercial streets full of workshops, people could watch endangered traditional trades such as papermaking, brewing, oil extraction and blacksmithing. Snack stalls offered a variety of delicacies typical of this region south of the Yangtze, such as ginger candy, rice cake and firm or silken tofu. The melodious shouts of street vendors in the morning drew people to this area. Here, you could witness the vicissitudes of life under the Republic of China, and appreciate the many flourishing scenes of professionals and tradesmen at work. These childhood experiences would remain with Tu Youyou throughout her life.

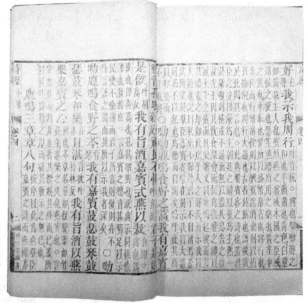

'Yo, yo, cries a herd of deer that eat wormwood in the wilderness,' from **The Book of Songs**

Twenty minutes walk east of this area was another typical region of 1930s Ningbo — San Jiangkou. This is the place where the Yao river, flowing from north to south, and the Fenghua river from south to north, join the Yong river. The waters then flow into the East China Sea via the estuary of Zhaobao mountain in Zhenhai district. At that time, Ningbo had commercial connections with nearly half of the country. In addition, trade at Jiangxia wharf in San Jiangkou had long been prosperous, with many ships calling there and transporting cargo to and from many destinations. This gave rise to the once popular saying: "Nowhere is better than Jiangxia, Ningbo."

However, in Tu's memory of her childhood, the flourishing trade scene at the wharf was not as attractive as Tianyi pavilion, less than two kilometers from her home.

Ningbo residents had always been proud of the city's abundant collection of books from down the years as well as its booming trade with all continents. For them, the classics of its urban civilization stored in the Tianyi pavilion mattered more than any material wealth generated by the port.

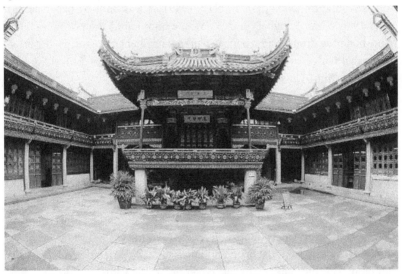

Tianyi pavilion, constructed in the middle of Ming dynasty, is the oldest existing private library in China, the longest surviving library in Asia and one of the three earliest-built family libraries in the world

Tianyi pavilion is an ancient library located west of Moon Lake. It has become a Ningbo landmark due to it being the oldest existing private library in China, the longest surviving library in Asia and one of the three earliest-built family libraries in the world.

Here in Tianyi pavilion, one can stroke the columns that line the aisles, explore the green courtyards and be surrounded by the literary atmosphere; one could also imagine the hardships involved in preserving and transmitting Chinese culture. Tianyi pavilion inherited the torch of Chinese traditional culture by recording history and enriching the lives of future generations. Here, visitors could appreciate the extensive and profound knowledge of Confucianism, Buddhism and Taoism.

Growing up in a place near Ningbo's most famous landmarks, Tu Youyou's memories of life on Kaiming Road were undoubtedly full of Ningbo flavor.

The Yao residence on 26 Kaiming Road, her maternal grandmother's house, evoked another important element of her childhood memories.

The house is the last surviving building on this road that dates from the Republic of China period (1912–1949). It was built by her maternal grandfather, Yao Yongbai. In a city with a tradition of respecting teachers and honoring truth, Yao Yongbai worked in Shanghai as a professor at Shanghai University of Political Science and Law, Fudan University and the Great China University.

The building faces south and consists of a reception room, lobby, central area and private rooms towards the rear. The reception room and lobby are in a two-story building comprising three rooms and two corridors. The building is decorated with wooden rails and the end panels are engraved with curling grass patterns. The main, single-story building contains three rooms and one alley, and is supported by five columns. The gable wall is decorated in the shape of five ponies. The back rooms are situated in a single-story flush gable roof building comprising three rooms and one alley. Across the empty lobby, there is a small and comfortable yard. A tall tree cloaks part of the main building with its luxuriant foliage. In early autumn, its leaves fall quietly and cover the whole yard.

In 1937, Japan launched a full-scale war of aggression against China. Four years later, Ningbo became an enemy-occupied area. The war forced the Tu family to move to the Yao residence, and Tu Youyou continued to live there until 1951, when she went to university.

Several celebrities used to live in buildings adjacent to the Yao residence, including Yuan Jue, 'the most famous scholar in Yongshang', Li Jingdi, a prominent local businessman, and Sun Chuanzhe, a famous stamp designer. The region was a gathering place for scholars and distinguished families.

Before Tu Youyou rose to prominence, the most famous figure in the Yao residence was Yao Qingsan, a renowned economist and Tu Youyou's uncle.

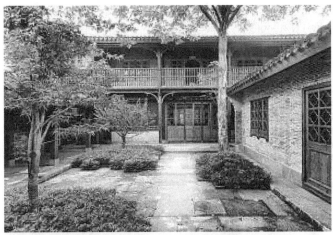

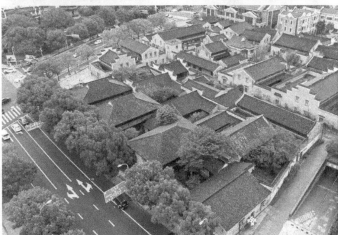

The Yao residence at 26 Kaiming Road, constructed by her maternal grandfather, Yao Yongbai. Tu Youyou lived there from the age of 11 until she started university. The top picture is the Yao residence; the one below is a panoramic view of the Yao residence

Yao Qingsan was born in 1911 and graduated from Fudan University in 1929. He went to study in France at the University of Paris's department of economics and politics. He then returned to China and worked in the general administration division of Shanghai Transportation Bank in 1931, becoming engaged in the study of the Chinese currency. In 1934, his study *Theories on Finance and Modern Currency Trends* was published as one of the earliest textbooks on finance in China.

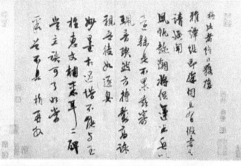

An example of the handwriting of Yuan Jue (1266-1327). He was an educational officer and lecturer at an academy in the Yuan dynasty (1271-1368), and was a leader of the literary world in the early Yuan dynasty

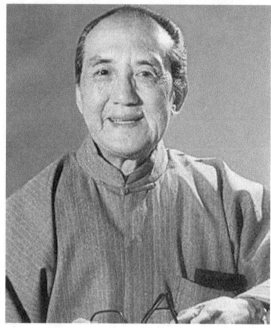

Sun Chuanzhe, one of China's most prominent stamp designers

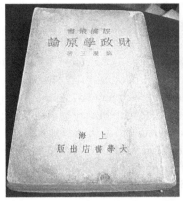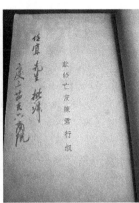

Theories on Finance *by Yao Qingsan*

In June 1934, the US Congress passed the Silver Purchase Act which increased the international price of silver and led to a large outflow of the precious metal from China. The Nanjing national government levied an export tax on silver, but the problem was still unresolved. A wide discussion ensued among economists and financiers about the silver problem and currency system reform. Ma Yinchu, an economist who was against the currency reforms, debated with supporters who were represented by Yao Qingsan and other scholars.

It was not until November 1935 that the advice of Yao and many other scholars was adopted and the currency reforms were put into effect. The reform was a key step in the modernization of China's currency system.

Yao Qingsan also had some connections with John Maynard Keynes, the famous British economist. It was Yao who introduced Keynes' thinking to China and he wrote the first analytical papers on his theories.

From 1953, Yao Qingsan began to work at the Hong Kong branch of Xinhua Bank. He was transferred to China Construction Financial (Hong Kong) in 1979 and worked there until 1985. Bank of China Group in Hong Kong grew out of these two organizations. Between the ages of 42 and 75, Yao Qingsan made great contributions to China's overseas finance development. He also introduced Tu Youyou's father to the world of banking.

Tu Youyou revered her successful maternal uncle and admired him as a role model all her life.

Educational Beginnings of the Tu Family

In line with Ningbo's tradition of highly valuing education, Tu Youyou's parents arranged for her to be sent to school. Despite being a girl, Tu Youyou was given the opportunity to receive an education, which reflected the importance her parents placed on the education of all their children.

In 1935, the five-year-old Tu Youyou was sent to a kindergarten by her parents. One year later, she entered Chongde private primary school in Ningbo to complete her studies from grade one to grade three. From grade four to grade six, she attended Maoxi private primary school. When she was 13 years old, she attended Qizhen private middle school in Ningbo, before being transferred to the private girls' school, Yongjiang Middle, at the age of 15.

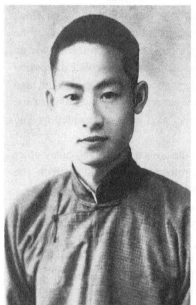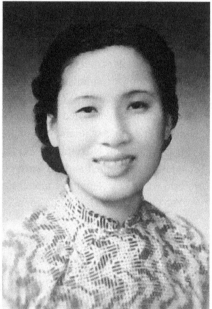

Tu Youyou's father Tu Liangui and her mother Yao Zhongqian

Some of the older locals regarded her as 'a delicate and pretty Ningbo girl with glasses and braids'.

Tu Youyou's father, Tu Liangui, was born in 1903, 29 years into the reign of Emperor Guangxu of the Qing dynasty. Nine years later, the Qing dynasty came to an end. As a consequence, Tu Liangui, one of the 20th generation of Tus, was among the first pupils to take advantage of a new trend in Ningbo of receiving a westernized education. After graduating from the first advanced primary school in Yin county, he attended Xiaoshi middle school. As for his children, Tu Liangui arranged a similar education; his three sons all acquired a decent education, and so did Tu Youyou, even though she was a girl.

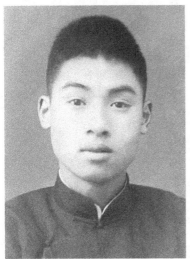 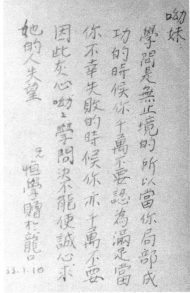

Tu Youyou's brother gave this photo of himself to his 14-year-old sister. The words written on the back of the photo are: 'Youyou, knowledge is infinite. Never be content with only partial success. Never be discouraged when you suffer setbacks. Youyou, knowledge never disappoints the one who sincerely pursues it'

However, the school years were interrupted in 1946 when the 16-year-old Tu Youyou endured a challenging ordeal: she was infected with tuberculosis and had to leave school. The Tus fell into straitened circumstances as a result of the war and Youyou's illness. It's not difficult to imagine the impact tuberculosis could have on such a young child; it was a challenge simply to survive. Fortunately, after more than two years of treatment and nursing care, Tu Youyou recovered and continued with her studies. Indeed, she says the experience was the origin of her interest in medicine and pharmacology. "Traditional Chinese medicines have magical effects. I thought at the time that I could keep myself free from disease and save other people's lives if I learned medicine and pharmacology. Why not do it?"

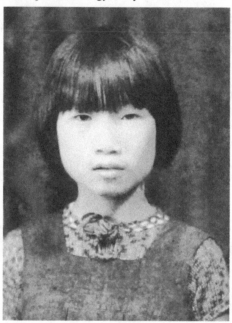

A young Tu Youyou

The spark that would lead her to become a famous pharmacologist came from this simple desire to cure herself and save the lives of others.

Over time, Tu Youyou's family stimulated her interest in medicine and pharmacology. Her father, Tu Liangui, was a bank clerk, but he took great pleasure in reading in his leisure time. The attic room that held numerous ancient books served as his study and it was also Tu Youyou's favorite place. When he read books there, she sat beside him pretending to read; she couldn't understand the text but most of the Chinese medicine books had illustrations. She enjoyed leafing through her father's books in those simple and happy days.

As the only daughter in her family, she was dearly loved by her parents. She liked eating sea snails, so her mother had some pickled and arranged for them to be taken to her during busy school days, which made many of her classmates envious.

A High School Student, Good at Biology

In 1948, having spent two years recovering from tuberculosis, the 18 year-old Tu Youyou attended Xiaoshi private middle school in Ningbo, the same school that her father attended.

Xiaoshi middle school was famous locally. It was established in February 1912 by the early Chinese physicist He Yujie, the local businessman Li Jingdi, and a number of famous Chinese scientists, such as Ye Bingliang, Cheng Xunzheng and Qian Baohang. The school strived to "secure funding and resources from private individuals, seek truth in education, and cultivate talent to enable the establishment of a government by the people". When it was founded, the school's stated philosophy was: "The value of education lies in its relevance, adapting to the needs of individuals, inheriting the school's fine traditions and keeping pace with the times."

The school shot to fame in 1917. Famous universities such as Fudan and St John's in Shanghai signed contracts with Xiaoshi middle school. According to these contracts, all graduates from Xiaoshi could be admitted to these universities without taking an exam.

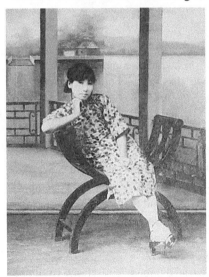

Tu Youyou's mother Yao Zhongqian in May 1929

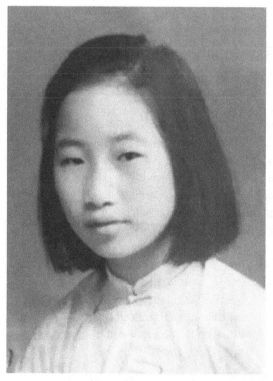

A young Tu Youyou

In February 1948, when Tu Youyou attended Xiaoshi middle school with an education that qualified her to start high school, the school was still recovering from the trauma of war that had concluded just three years earlier. It was not until October 25, 1945 that Xiaoshi was reinstituted after the fall of Ningbo in April 1941. So October 25 was set as the anniversary of the founding of Xiaoshi middle school.

Xiaoshi middle school, whose motto is 'Patriotic, Progressive, Scientific, Practical', can boast an impressive alumni group. To date, 15 members of the Chinese Academy of Sciences (CAS) and the Chinese Academy of Engineering graduated from the school, which can be ranked nationally alongside Nankai middle school in Tianjin, and the Fourth middle school and Huiwen middle school in Beijing.

Ningbo's Xiaoshi middle school educated three scientists who would be

14

elected to the CAS in 1955: scientist Ji Yufeng studied in the school's third year, in 1916; experimental embryologist Tong Dizhou graduated from the school in the ninth year, in 1922; and soil agricultural chemist Li Qingkui studied its high school department in 1930. In 1980, another five graduates from Xiaoshi were elected as members of the CAS, including geophysicist Weng Wenbo, soil chemist Zhu Zuxiang, breeding geneticist Bao Wenkui, nuclear physicist Dai Chuanzeng and medical scientist Chen Zhongwei. In 1955, five Xiaoshi middle school graduates became academicians of the CAS and members of the Chinese Academy of Engineering: the materials scientist Xu Zuyao, Chen Jingxiong, specializing in electromagnetic and microwave technology, Mao Yongze, who worked in the field of nuclear technology, the inorganic chemical expert Zhou Guangyao, and the nuclear engineering expert Hu Side. In 1997, another two Xiaoshi graduates, the specialist in electronic information systems engineering Tong Zhipeng, and the expert in civil structural engineering and protective engineering Chen Zhaozhong, were elected to the Chinese Academy of Engineering.

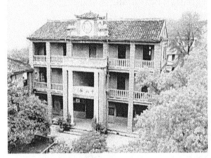

Xiaoshi middle school's Zhongshan Hall

These 15 academicians educated by Xiaoshi middle school are a testimony to Ningbo's reputation as the 'hometown of academicians'.

Despite attending this famous school, Tu Youyou's overall performance during high school was not outstanding. According to the school's student records, Tu Youyou, student number A342, obtained an average score of 71.25 for Chinese, 71.5 for English, 70 for math, 80.5 for biology and 67.5 for chemistry.

Her excellent performance in the biology exam was due to her strong interest in the subject. She always listened to her biology teacher with great interest. Once, the teacher joked: "If the other students were as diligent and attentive as Tu Youyou, I'd be happy, no matter how hard my job."

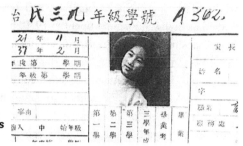

An extract from Tu Youyou's senior high school file

As Tu Youyou herself admitted: "I was quiet and humble then." Her middle school classmate, Chen Xiaozhong, concurred: "She was humble and plainly dressed. She was not conspicuous, and she was mostly silent."

In addition to studying at the school, Tu Youyou had another important connection with Xiaoshi middle school. Li Tingzhao was in the year below and at the time there was little communication between the two students. Certainly, they would not have anticipated getting married in future.

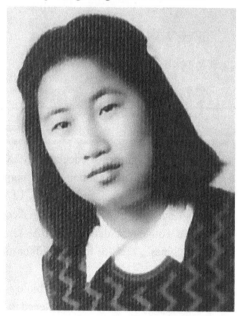

Tu Youyou in senior high school, 1950

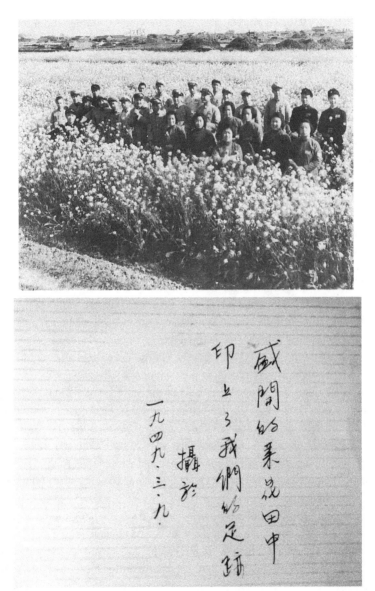

On March 9, 1949, Tu Youyou took a series of photos with her classmates in nearby fields. The words on the back of this photo read: 'Our footprints are left in fields of blooming flowers'

In March 1950, Tu Youyou transferred to Ningbo middle school for her third year of high school, which was also her last school year in Ningbo. Her classroom teacher at the time, Xu Jizi, wrote the following words to encourage this humble student: "Don't be content with a peaceful life. Have the courage to face challenges."

It should be noted that many outstanding students graduated from Ningbo middle school along with Tu Youyou in 1951, including the former executive vice-president of Peking University Wang Yizun, the academician of the CAS Shi Zhongci, and the famous publisher Fu Xuancong.

In the summer of 1951, after graduating from high school, Tu Youyou was determined to continue her academic career. Therefore, winning a university place became her new goal.

When submitting her applications before the examination, the independently minded Tu Youyou applied to the pharmacy department of the medical college at Peking University. At that time, few universities in China had such a department, so the pharmacy department at the medical college in Peking University was a bellwether. Tu Youyou's choice of subject was quite unusual since there was no history of studying medicine in the Tu family. In fact, Tu Youyou had yearned for this opportunity since becoming infected with tuberculosis. Why did she choose to study pharmacy? In her opinion, medicines were crucial in the treatment of diseases.

At that time, the new China had not yet introduced national college entrance examinations, in which setting questions, testing and enrollment are administered in a unified way. The country was still divided into six test regions – the northeast, north, northwest, east, central south and southwest. Enrollment was conducted by the colleges and universities from the same region. Famous universities, such as Peking University and Tsinghua, belonged to the north region.

According to the regulations, as a student from Zhejiang province with an ambition to study in the north, Tu Youyou had to leave for the provincial capital, Hangzhou, in order to sit the exam. This meant saying goodbye to her hometown of Ningbo, where she had lived for more than 20 years. Over three days of tests, the 20-year-old Tu Youyou completed the college entrance examination at a venue in Zhejiang University.

During that period, the admission lists of universities in the north region would be published in newspapers such as *People's Daily* and *Guangming Daily*. Therefore, while waiting for the results, Tu Youyou got into the habit of reading these newspapers from time to time.

At the end of the summer of 1951, Tu Youyou received a letter of admission from Peking University. She embarked on her journey to Beijing in north China, where she started her higher education.

She said that, as a girl, she was "very lucky" to continue her studies in university at a time when socialist construction was just starting to be implemented. Women began to have the opportunity to 'go outside' for the first time in order to develop their intelligence and wisdom. The fact that Tu Youyou was among the first intake of female college students in the new China reflected women's irreplaceable role in the construction and development of the country.

Chapter 2

Embarking on the Road Towards Learning Medicine

School Life in Peking University

In 1951, three years after the founding of the new China, Tu Youyou was admitted to the school of pharmacy in Peking University as one of the country's most brilliant talents.

In the 1950s, the university's medical school had a distinctively western flavor in this ancient city with a history of thousands of years. The university, located near the Xishiku cathedral in Beijing's Xicheng district, was surrounded by ancient buildings that were part of the royal palace complex in imperial times. However, the students' first sight was always a classic Gothic building, the Xishiku cathedral. The old site was replaced by the first outpatient department of the Oral Medicine Hospital of Peking University. During the period of their study in university, the laboratories and dormitories of Tu Youyou and her classmates were located at No. 13 Caiyuan Hutong.

According to Zhou Shikun, Tu Youyou's classmate and chief pharmacist at the Beijing Health Vocational College, their class was known as the eighth class according to the year of enrollment. There were 70 to 80 students in the class. Zhou Shikun, the same age as Tu Youyou, recalled that they were older than the other students, by as much as three years in one case.

On entering their fourth year, the class was classified into the three majors – drug testing, pharmaceutical chemistry and pharmacognosy. Forty students chose pharmaceutical chemistry, accounting for the largest percentage, while 12 students, including Tu Youyou, chose pharmacognosy, accounting for the smallest percentage.

Pharmacognosy is the study of traditional Chinese medicinal materials derived from plants, animals or minerals that are either unprocessed or only lightly processed.

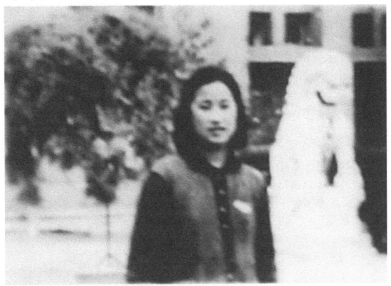

Tu Youyou wearing the school badge of Peking University, 1952

Wang Muzou, who would later become a researcher in the pharmaceutical department of the Academy of Medical Science of China, was in the same year as Tu Youyou and chose the same major. He said that, at that time, most graduates majoring in pharmacognosy were later engaged in research, while graduates majoring in pharmaceutical chemistry would go on to work for large pharmaceutical companies nationwide.

Although the students were classified into different majors, they took the courses together, albeit with a different emphasis in majors. Tu Youyou, majoring in pharmacognosy, had more classes in this subject than the other specialized courses. The main contents of her course were classifying and identifying TCM and observing their internal structures by using microscopic sections.

The pharmacognosy course was taken by Professor Lou Zhicen, who got his PhD in Britain before returning to China in 1951, when he was the only professor majoring in pharmacognosy. Later, he would become a pioneer of modern pharmacognosy in China and president of the Chinese Pharmaceutical Association (CPA).

The pharmacy department also offered other important specialized courses, including pharmaceutical chemistry and botanical chemistry. Botanical chemistry was taught by Professor Lin Qishou, who had studied in the US. His lectures, mainly about extracting and separating efficacious ingredients in plants, studying their chemical properties, identifying their chemical structures and writing the methods of chemical identification, also covered the selection of different extracting agents in the process of extracting effective components.

The fundamental knowledge of the pharmacognosy course and the methodology used in the botanical chemistry course would become important parts of Tu Youyou's later work.

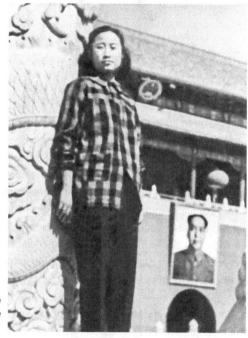

Tu Youyou in Tiananmen Square when she was a college student, 1954

In the early years of the new China, many aspects of society were underdeveloped. In the medical field, there was a lack of both medicine and medical staff. As qualified medical workers were badly needed in

China, many students competed to apply to the medical colleges, in which pharmaceutical chemistry in the pharmacy department was the most popular major at the time.

However, young Tu Youyou was interested in pharmacognostics, an 'unpopular' major at the time. She selected the subject as her major rather than follow the trend, and then she put it into practice throughout her working life. Whenever she was asked if she had ever doubted her decision, she answered that it was the wisest choice she had ever made, and that she had no regrets.

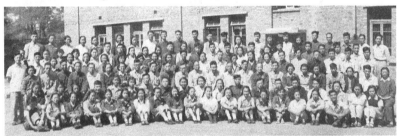

The staff and students of the pharmacy department of Peking University Health Science Center in September 1955. Tu Youyou is seventh from left in the back row. Ninth left in the third row is Lin Qishou, a phytochemist whose most outstanding achievement is a Chinese medicinal herb chemical book written in the 1970s, which is the only systematic and complete study on phytochemistry in China; 10th from left in the third row is Lou Zhicen, a pharmacognosist, deputy director of the pharmacy department at Peking University Health Science Center, one of the first group of academicians in the department of medicine and health engineering, and the academic leader in the key discipline of pharmocognosy in China; 11th from left in the third row is Jiang Mingqian, an organic chemist and department member of the CAS; 12th from left in the third row is Xue Yu, pharmaceutical chemist, director of the pharmacy department at the medical school of National Peking University; 13th from left in the third row is Wang Xu, organic chemist, academician of the CAS, director of the pharmacy department at Peking University Health Science Center

The Love Story of a Junior Research Fellow

In 1955, after four years' hard work, Tu Youyou graduated from Peking University.

It was a time when many important institutions were on the cusp of being developed. The Academy of Traditional Chinese Medicine directly attached to the Ministry of Public Health, which is today known as the China Academy of Chinese Medical Science (CACMS), began to prepare for its establishment. A group of famous veteran doctors of TCM who were elected from different regions were sent to Beijing in order to strengthen Chinese medicine research. Having just graduated from university and being full of energy, Tu Youyou was assigned to work in the Pharmaceutical Research Institute of the Academy of TCM.

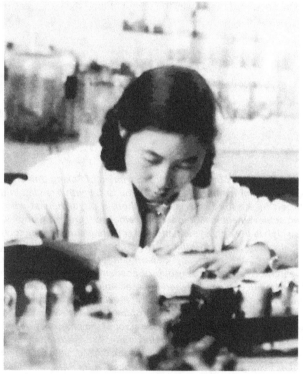

In 1955, Tu Youyou was assigned to the Academy of Chinese Medicine, part of the Ministry of Public Health (now known as CACMS)

At the beginning, Tu Youyou was mainly engaged in pharmacognosy. In 1956, great progress was being made in the prevention and treatment of schistosomiasis, an infection caused by a parasitic worm that lives in fresh water in subtropical and tropical regions. Tu and her college teacher, Lou Zhicen, successfully completed research into an effective medicine, derived from the flowering plant Chinese Lobelia. The research findings were recorded in *TCM Identification Reference Materials* published by People's Medical Publishing House in 1958. Later on, Tu Youyou finished her research into starwort, a plant that comes in various types and which is used in TCM, and the findings were included in *Chinese Traditional Medicine Records* in 1959. The two studies on Chinese Lobelia and starwort were components of Tu's university major.

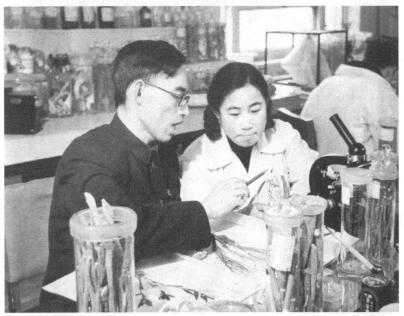

In the 1950s, Lou Zhicen, an associate professor, tutored Tu Youyou in researching Chinese medicine when Tu was a research assistant at the Pharmaceutical Research Institute of the China Academy of TCM, part of the Ministry of Public Health

Like many other scientific researchers, Tu Youyou paid little attention to her personal life. She threw herself into her work and never cared much for herself. Once, she couldn't find her ID card and she asked her colleagues to help look for it. They opened her suitcase and found everything inside in a terrible mess. "She's not like a girl, as girls can't be so careless," they joked.

Now, Tu Youyou pledged to put her everyday affairs in order: "I'm still

25

not good at household duties," she said, "and my husband Older Li [Li Tingzhao] always bought the vegetables and did the shopping after we were married."

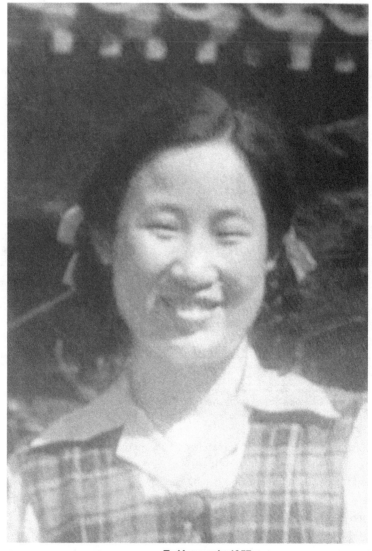

Tu Youyou in 1957

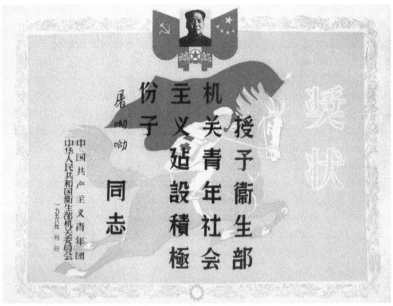

In 1958, Tu Youyou was granted the title of Young Activist of Socialist Construction by the Institute of the Ministry of Health

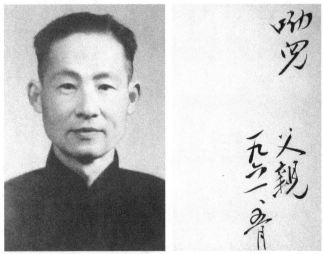

In 1961, Tu Youyou's father gave her a photo with the following inscription on the back: 'To Youyou... father, May 1961'

27

Li Tingzhao was born in September 1931 in Ningbo, Tu Youyou's hometown. They were classmates in Xiaoshi middle school. In 1951, after graduating from this school, Li Tingzhao went to Beijing Foreign Language School. During the period of the War to Resist US Aggression and Aid Korea, Li Tingzhao and many of his classmates proposed to go to the Korean battlefield. Hearing their proposals, Premier Zhou Enlai said: "You had better continue your study in China since the country badly needs talented people like you." Therefore, Li Tingzhao stayed and continued his study in cram school at China Agriculture University. At that time, he wanted to apply to the Beijing Institute of Technology or Tsinghua University; in 1952, he was successful in his attempt to be admitted to the former. At university, he excelled academically. From 1954 to 1960, he was sent to study abroad at the Leningrad Technological Institute in the Soviet Union, where he obtained his master's degree. After returning to China, Li was assigned to work in Beiman steel plant, located in Qiqihar, Heilongjiang province. He later worked at Ma'anshan Iron and Steel (1961-1964), Beijing Iron and Steel Research Institute (1964-1976) and the State Department of Metallurgy, among other places. From working in a steel plant to being engaged in scientific research and management, he was tightly bound to steel.

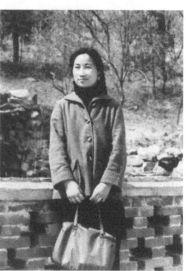

Tu Youyou, in the block release TCM training class for doctors of western medicine at the Academy of TCM, 1962

While working at Ma'anshan Iron and Steel in Ma'anshan, one of his sisters happened to be living in Beijing. Tu Youyou often went to visit Li Tingzhao's sister because they were both from Ningbo. Therefore, Li Tingzhao often met his classmate Tu Youyou when he visited his sister in Beijing. His sister sensed a mutual affection between them and actively acted as a matchmaker. As time passed, the two hearts gradually became one.

In 1963, two years after their reunion in Beijing, they got married.

Their friends joked that the marriage of Tu Youyou and Li Tingzhao was the integration of tradition (TCM) and modernity (steel).

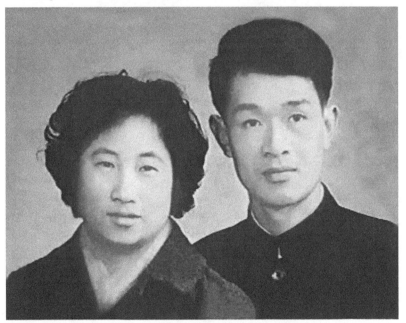

Tu Youyou and Li Tingzhao when they were young

Wang Muzou's wife was also acquainted with Tu Youyou. She said Tu was not good at housework, with almost all the household duties performed by her husband. "Different from other girls, she is broad-minded and dedicates herself to work," she said.

Although Tu Youyou and Li Tingzhao played different roles in their family, they had the same focus − devotion.

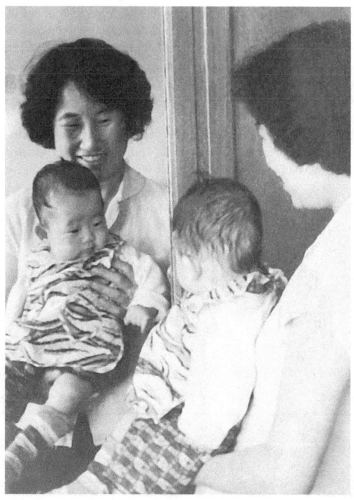

Young mother Tu Youyou and her elder daughter Li Min in the summer of 1965

"It was most important to us at that time to fulfill the tasks assigned by the state. We left our children for the duration of a task." Tu Youyou was calm when she talked about the past. At that time in the late 1960s, she was sent to Hainan, and Li Tingzhao, who once studied metallurgy in the Soviet Union, was sent to the May 7 Cadre School in Yunnan province. In order to properly finish their work, they made the painful decision to send their elder daughter, not yet four years old, to a boarding nursery school while their younger daughter was cared for by their parents in Ningbo. According to Tu Youyou, the prolonged separation from her parents meant that "our elder daughter was unwilling to call us mum and dad when we brought her home." Their younger daughter Li Jun recalls that she didn't have a clear impression of her mother until the age of three.

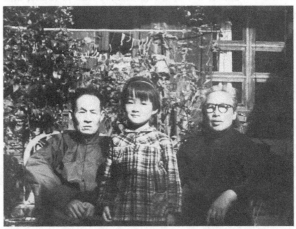

A photo of Tu Youyou's parents and her younger daughter Li Jun, taken in the spring of 1974. In order to properly finish 'Mission 523', a top-secret government unit that was formed to find a cure for malaria, Tu Youyou sent Li Jun to Ningbo and entrusted her parents to look after her

A few years after Li Jun was sent to Ningbo, Tu Youyou spared some time out of her busy scientific research to visit the daughter she yearned for day and night. On that day, Li Jun stood at the gate of her grandparent's house, seeing someone with luggage walking towards her quickly with open arms, crying: "Little Jun, Little Jun."

However, Li Jun unconsciously stepped back. At that moment, she had no memories of her mother. She didn't know that this woman before her was Tu Youyou, the mother she had imagined so many times. Li Jun still wonders now how her mother recognized her.

For a long time, they only saw each other once every three to four years, and Li Jun couldn't understand why her mother had left her family, and particularly her children, for the sake of her career in scientific research.

Thinking about those 'strange' mother-and-daughter meetings, Tu

Youyou had doubts about her decision. Many years later, she still lamented: "When my daughter grew up, she didn't want to come back to Beijing to live with us."

Today, such a choice can seem heartless. However, for a couple whose love for their daughters and granddaughters is evident in the many family photos about their home, it was a choice they had to make, and one that people at that time could understand.

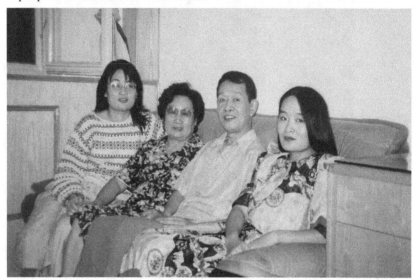

A family photo taken in 1996. From left to right: the elder daughter Li Min, Tu Youyou, Li Tingzhao and the younger daughter Li Jun

Taking a Block Release Class to Learn TCM

In 1959, while she had been in the job for four years, Tu Youyou attended session three of a block release class for doctors of Western medicine to learn TCM at the Academy of TCM, organized by the Ministry of Health. Since then, she started to systematically study the subject of TCM.

This experience paved the way for Tu Youyou to seek inspiration from TCM and then to discover artemisinin.

In the 1950s and 1960s, it had become common practice for TCM to learn from western medicine.

In 1954, Chairman Mao Zedong, with great foresight, proposed that "western medicine learn from TCM" for national health systems and advocated the combination of traditional Chinese and western medicine. His aim was to create a new medicine that could draw on the advantages of both systems to contribute to the construction of the new China. To this end, Mao put forward a comprehensive and profound direction: "In future, the focus is to encourage western medicine to learn from TCM." He also implemented some specific improvement measures, sending 100-200 graduates from medical universities and colleges to learn clinical experience from famous doctors of TCM. A modest approach facilitates learning from others, according to Mao, and it's an honor for western medicine to learn from TCM. With learning, education and improvement, the boundary between the two traditions will be broken and a new medicine will be developed to contribute to the world.

At that time, the idea of 'western medicine learning from TCM' was less common than it is today.

After the foundation of the new China, the national health situation was grave: the country was stricken with epidemic disease outbreaks, medicine shortages and poor medical conditions. There were only about 20,000 doctors of western medicine nationwide. And while there were more than 100,000 practitioners of TCM, they didn't play their roles properly.

At that time, TCM failed to play an important role because of the number of impractical and harsh provisions contained in traditional Chinese management documents, such as *Provisional Regulations on Doctors of TCM, Implementation Rules for Provisional Regulations on Doctors of TCM* and *Provisional Regulations on Examinations for Doctors, Doctors of TCM, Dentists and Pharmacists.*

One of the results was that, in 1953, there were only 14,000 doctors of TCM who were registered and qualified in 92 large and medium-sized cities and 165 counties. In 18 counties in the Yuncheng region of Shanxi province, for example, there was not a single qualified doctor of TCM. The level of TCM in Tianjin was relatively high but, out of more than 530 doctors of TCM who took the TCM qualification exam in 1953, only 55 passed. In 1950 and 1951, Jiangxi provincial health department examined practitioners of TCM and either struck them off or issued them with long-term or temporary licenses based on their performance. A total of 8,728 doctors in Jiangxi were registered; 424 doctors were recognized as formal doctors of TCM; 3,648 doctors were appraised as temporary doctors of TCM; the remaining doctors were actually disqualified from practicing medicine. In 1950, the 1,355 unqualified doctors were asked to take an exam set by the prefectural commissioner's office. However, as a request made by many doctors to 'postpone the exam' was rejected, only 727 doctors took the exam and 327 of them failed, causing discontent among many doctors of TCM.

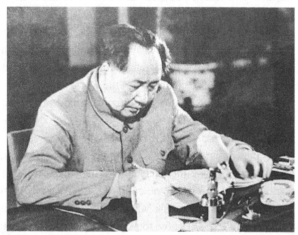

Mao Zedong in the 1950s

In addition, there were problems in specific aspects of the health care system. For instance, the role of TCM was not taken into account in the implementation of the socialized medicine system. The costs of TCM couldn't be reimbursed and major hospitals didn't accept doctors of TCM. Continuation schools for doctors of TCM were set up to introduce the simple diagnosis and treatment techniques of western medicine and encourage doctors of TCM to learn western medicine. Medical colleges and universities declined to offer TCM courses; the Chinese Medical Association didn't receive members of TCM; the production, supply and marketing of traditional Chinese medicinal materials lacked effective management; and some patented Chinese medicines that were popular with the public and proven to cure diseases were banned without reason. Articles were published claiming that TCM was 'feudal medicine' and argued that it should be eliminated along with feudal society in general.

On August 24, 1956, Mao Zedong received representatives participating in the first national music week and had a conversation with the director of the Chinese Musicians Association. During the conversation, he explained in depth why 'Sinicization' was necessary, and frequently illustrated it with the example of "the combination of TCM and western medicine". He went on: "A doctor could quickly understand TCM if he had learned western medicine, anatomy, pharmacology, etc. before researching TCM and its materials. We must clarify the essential principles that foreign fundamentals should be learned. And it is unreasonable to use only the Chinese scalpel. For medical science, modern western science shall be applied to research the laws of TCM… You are 'doctors of western medicine', but you need to Sinicize what you have learned and research Chinese medicine with what you have learned… You should draw on the advantages of western medicine to improve Chinese medicine, thus creating something exclusive to China with a unique national style. This is the reasonable way in which national confidence will not be lost."

Mao Zedong had clearly and fully expressed his thoughts on "the combination of TCM and western medicine". This meant encouraging doctors of western medicine to learn from doctors of TCM, inspire doctors of TCM to learn modern science and technology, closely combine TCM and western medicine, and inherit and carry forward TCM through the application of modern science and technology to create a new development road of medicine and pharmacology with Chinese characteristics.

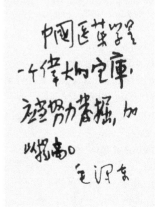

The important instruction made by Mao Zedong in October 1958, on the Summary Report on the Block Release Class for Doctors of Western Medicine to Learn TCM, *delivered by the Ministry of Health to the central government*

On October 11, 1958, the Ministry of Health prepared the *Summary Report on the Block Release Study Class for Doctors of Western Medicine to Learn TCM*, and Mao Zedong gave his famous instruction that "TCM is a great treasure that shall be fully explored and improved". It showed that Mao Zedong regarded Chinese medicine as a precious heritage bestowed by Chinese traditional culture with special stress on fully exploiting its practical value.

Ever since then, the combination of Chinese and western medicine gained momentum.

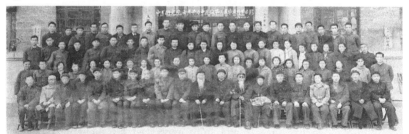

Graduates in the block release class (third session) in 1960 for doctors of western medicine to study TCM at the Academy of TCM, organized by the Ministry of Health. Sixth from left in the second row is Tu Youyou; eighth from right in the front row is Pu Fuzhou, the outstanding therapist of his time who was the primary care doctor of Premier Zhou Enlai; 10th from right in the front row is Du Ziming, an expert in TCM Chinese bone-setting, who was visited on his death bed at the Friendship Hospital by Premier Zhou; 10th from left in the front row is Gao Henian, then vice-president of the Academy of TCM; first from left in the front row is Tang Youzhi, master of TCM who once cured Mao Zedong of an eye disease; 10th from right in the fourth row is Gao Xiaoshan, senior researcher and a pioneer of medicinal property theories

In this important instruction on Chinese medicine, Mao Zedong stressed: "If two-year block release classes with 70-80 student doctors of western medicine were set up in each province, city and autonomous region in 1958, by winter 1960 or spring 1961 there would be about 2,000 senior doctors with knowledge of both TCM and western medicine, some of whom might become outstanding theorists."

According to data collected in 1960 by a national meeting designed to exchange the experiences of western medicine and TCM, there were 37 block release classes involving more than 2,300 students and 36,000 doctors being taught TCM during this period. Many prominent and intermediate medical colleges offered courses in TCM, cultivating a group of doctors trained in western medicine who were learning TCM. They went on to become experts in that field and academic leaders in TCM and in combined TCM and western medicine.

In 1959, Tu Youyou became an active member of the third session of block release classes for doctors of western medicine to learn TCM at the Academy of TCM. After studying for two-and-a-half years in the block release class, she gained both theoretical knowledge and clinical learning.

On the basis of her major, Tu Youyou visited medicine enterprises to learn TCM identification and processing techniques from experienced pharmaceutical staff. She was also involved in processing medicine in Beijing. Through all this, she furthered her knowledge of the varieties, authentication, quality and processing techniques of medicine.

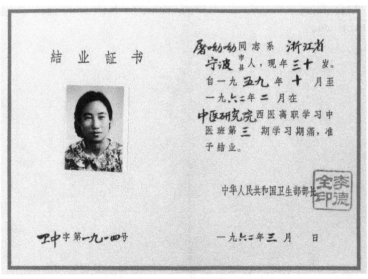

For two-and-a-half years, Tu Youyou attended the block release class for doctors of western medicine at the Academy of TCM, organized by the Ministry of Health. This is her 1962 course completion certificate

Processing is a special pharmaceutical feature of TCM, involving dispensing, preparation and clinical application, based on the properties of medicine materials and TCM theory. Chinese medicine can only be used after processing. Toxicity and side effects can be reduced and eliminated, the properties of the medicine can be changed or moderated, and efficacy can be improved by means of cleansing, cutting and further processing.

After finishing her learning in the block release class, Tu Youyou participated in the research of TCM assigned by the Ministry of Health. She was one of the chief compilers of the *Summary of Experience in TCM Processing*. The book extensively summarized the experience in processing TCM from different Chinese provinces and cities and systematically catalogued the relevant literature.

Through this pioneering block release training, Tu Youyou was able to understand the literature of both TCM and western medicine, and grasped their differences in history and philosophy so as to combine the practical knowledge of traditional medicine and modern biomedicine at the highest level. Thus, she became one of the few outstanding theorists as expounded by Mao Zedong and laid a solid foundation for her future research into artemisinin.

Chapter 3

Persistence in the Discovery of Artemisinin

Mysterious '523'

January 21, 1969 was an important day for Tu Youyou, and one that changed her life.

On that day, she learned about a major national collaborative project – 'Project 523' – that she hadn't heard of before.

The director of the Project 523 office made a special visit to the Academy of TCM and remarked frankly: "Anti-malaria research using TCM has been conducted for years. In the past, researchers have investigated areas where malaria prevailed and collected and tested proven formulas. Certain effects have been shown, but none have been satisfactory. There are problems with usage, preparation and so on. Many formulas have been collected and most of them are complex. We don't know which medicines and formulas are better as we lack experience and knowledge of the methods. We hope you will join in this task."

Malaria was traditionally known as *dabaizi* in Chinese, the word being used to describe typical symptoms such as shaking. Today, malaria has almost been eradicated in China. Most people only see the disease in movies, television shows or literature set in times of war or in ancient days. People suffering from malaria alternately run a high fever and shiver with cold.

Malaria was also an invisible killer of soldiers. In world history, the disease has resulted in a sharp depletion in troop numbers, leading to military operation failures.

In the battle against malaria, the most effective first medicine was derived from the cinchona plant. In the 19th century, French chemists extracted the anti-malaria ingredient of quinine from cinchona bark. Later, scientists found an alternative to quinine in the form of chloroquine, which then became the leading medicine for treating malaria.

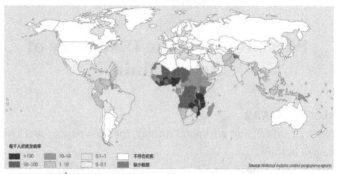

Countries and regions with malaria transmission in 2013

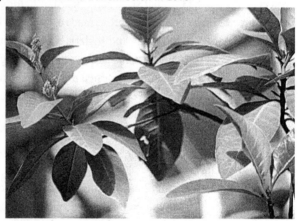

Cinchona leaves

However, after being controlled by chloroquine for nearly 200 years, plasmodium, a genus of parasitic protozoa that causes malaria, presented a strong resistance to these drugs. In the 1960s, malaria raged uncontrolled in Southeast Asia once again.

During this period, the US became embroiled in the Vietnam War, which involved more participants and had the most profound influence of any war since World War II. As the war escalated, the casualties rose on both the American and Vietnamese sides.

However, an enemy more terrible than bullets and bombs soon appeared during the war: drug-resistant malaria. The US and Vietnamese soldiers struggled in the tropical forests while malaria was like a third force assaulting the warring armies. According to official data, the US Army's non-combat loss of soldiers in 1964 was four to five times higher than the number of those killed in action. The morbidity of malaria among US troops stationed in Vietnam reached 50%. According to data compiled by the Hanoi Bureau of Health on the Vietnam People's Armed Forces from 1961 to 1968, the number of patients with noncombat-related illnesses far exceeded the number of wounded soldiers and most of them were suffering from malaria; the only exception was in the first quarter of 1968, when the number of wounded soldiers was higher.

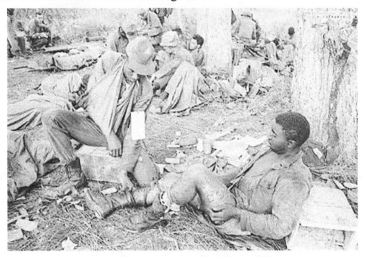

Soldiers threatened by malaria during the Vietnam War

Vietnam is a tropical country, with mountains and dense jungles. The climate is hot and humid. Mosquitoes and insects breed in all seasons, and malaria epidemics persisted throughout the year. Chloroquine and its derivatives became almost ineffective against the malaria that was prevalent in Vietnam.

A crucial advantage would be secured if the US or Vietnam could find a way to resist the disease.

In order to solve the problem, America set up a special malaria committee, increased research grants and organized dozens of units to conduct anti-malaria medicine research. By 1972, the Walter Reed Army Institute of Research had screened 214,000 compounds but had failed to find an ideal anti-malaria medicine with a new structure.

The general secretary of the Vietnam Communist Party Ho Chi Minh personally visited China to ask Mao Zedong for support in anti-malaria medicine and methods.

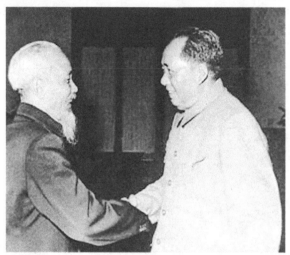

Mao Zedong receives the general secretary of the Vietnam Communist Party Ho Chi Minh, 1965

Having suffered from malaria himself during the Revolutionary War, Mao understood the harm it could cause. He said: "Solving your problem is solving ours."

At the request of Vietnam, Chairman Mao Zedong and Premier Zhou Enlai instructed relevant departments to set up a project for emergency aid and combat readiness tasks to deal with malaria in tropical zones, as the disease had seriously influenced the Viet Cong's fighting capacity and military operations. At that time, it was an important political task for medical scientists in the Chinese military to develop a new anti-malaria medicine. From 1964, research into anti-malaria medicine was conducted in the military. In 1966, experts from the Institute of Microbiology and Epidemiology and the Institute of Pharmacology and Toxicology of the

Academy of Military Medical Sciences conducted research into emergency prevention prescriptions and designed two types of anti-malaria pills, extending the prevention period from one week, to 10 days to two weeks.

In consideration of the urgency and difficulty of providing medicine to treat Plasmodium falciparum, one of the species of Plasmodium that cause malaria in humans, it was not realistic to complete the task within a short period by relying on military and scientific research alone. This task of emergency aid and combat readiness could be accomplished only by securing the involvement of domestic scientific researchers and promoting army-civilian cooperation. Therefore, the Academy of Military Medical Sciences of the People's Liberation Army (PLA) drafted a three-year research plan based on the prevention and treatment requirements of tropical drug-resistant falciparum malaria. The general logistics department of the PLA held discussions with the State Scientific and Technological Commission, the Ministry of Health, Ministry of Chemical Industry, State Commission of Science and Technology for the National Defense Industry, the CAS and the China National Pharmaceutical Industry Corporation. They were asked to organize their subordinate units of scientific research, medical treatment, teaching and pharmacy to jointly undertake these tasks based on an overall plan and mutual cooperation.

The State Scientific and Technological Commission and the general logistics department of the PLA held a collaborative meeting for research into medicine for the prevention and treatment of malaria on May 23, 1967 in Beijing. The meeting was attended by relevant ministries and commissions, leaders directly under the army headquarters and military leaders of relevant provinces, cities and districts along with their superior units. At the meeting, the three-year research plan was discussed and agreed.

Thus, research into new anti-malaria medicine began.

As the task was a confidential emergency military project for foreign aid and combat readiness, it was codenamed the '523' project because the meeting was held on May 23.

'523' became known to the public soon after Tu Youyou won the Nobel prize. Many people associated the number with research into artemisinin. In fact, as a large and confidential scientific research project, '523' involved

43

not only research into artemisinin but all aspects of malaria prevention and treatment. Many provinces, cities and industries were involved in the project.

The process of malaria prevention and treatment after 1949 can be divided into four stages. Stage one: investigation and the lowering of morbidity in the 1950s; stage two: the control of disease transmission in the 1960s and 1970s; stage three: the elimination of malaria in the 1980s and 1990s; stage four: consolidating achievements in malaria elimination after 2000.

Conducted in the 1960s and 1970s, the '523' project was part of stage two. It was not just aimed at 'resisting US aggression and aiding Vietnam'. In the 1950s, several planning schemes were launched, including the program for malaria prevention and treatment in minority areas. Health teams, epidemic prevention teams and medical teams were sent to hyperendemic areas of malaria to treat patients and conduct preventive work. Malaria dispensaries were established to conduct scientific research into malaria prevention and treatment and train technical experts. Malaria training classes were set up to train professional technical teams. With the implementation of this series of activities, the prevention and treatment of malaria in China came under systematic management and the incidence of malaria declined from 102.8 new cases per 10,000 in 1955 to 21.6 new cases per 10,000 in 1958.

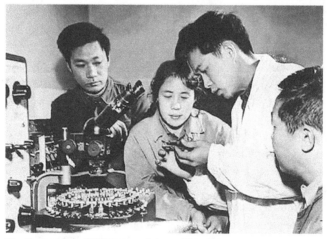

Members of the '523' research team at work

However, a large-scale outbreak of malaria occurred in China from the early 1960s to the early 1970s due to political, economic and natural factors. During this time, there were between 10m and 20m people suffering from malaria. Between 1960 and 1970, the national average incidence increased from 155.4 new cases per 10,000 to 296.1 per 10,000. The incidence rate in 1970 was the highest since 1949.

It seemed that Mao Zedong's expression "Solving your problem is solving ours" had profound implications. Malaria was an internal and external menace at that time and finding an immediate solution was imperative.

The purpose of the '523' project was clear: to develop malaria prevention and treatment medicine through civil-military cooperation. The medicine should be efficient, fast-acting and long-lasting.

After that, general investigation and screening studies into anti-malaria medicine were carried out in seven provinces and cities. By 1969, more than 10,000 compounds and Chinese herbal medicines including Artemisia annua had been screened, but no ideal results had been obtained.

Taking the Post of Research Group Leader

The Academy of TCM regarded being assigned the '523' project as a challenge. As the academy was severely impacted by the 'Cultural Revolution', the work of many experienced specialists was suspended, and scientific research was almost stopped.

Which individual was best able to undertake this important task?

The answer was the 39-year-old Tu Youyou. Although she was still a junior research fellow at the time, she had been working in the Institute of Chinese Materia Medica for 14 years. As a second-tier member of the institute, she was then undertaking research into the extraction of effective chemical components from plants, utilizing her knowledge of both TCM and western medicine.

At that time, Tu Youyou had the best qualities for this task at the Academy of TCM. Jiang Tingliang, a former director of the Institute of Chinese Materia Medica of the Academy of TCM who had worked with Tu Youyou since he was in his twenties, said that he assigned her the important project because she had solid knowledge of both TCM and western medicine and a scientific research capacity recognized by her colleagues.

Since January 1969, she had been a busy figure in the Institute of Chinese Materia Medica of the Academy of TCM, someone who was absorbed in reading numerous medical books of all dynasties, earnestly visiting veteran doctors of TCM, and even personally reading letters from the public.

Appointed as leader of the research group, the 39-year-old Tu Youyou embarked on her anti-malarial journey. No one expected the appointment would be the catalyst for the great progress of the '523' project.

At the very beginning, Tu Youyou led the project on her own, without any assistants.

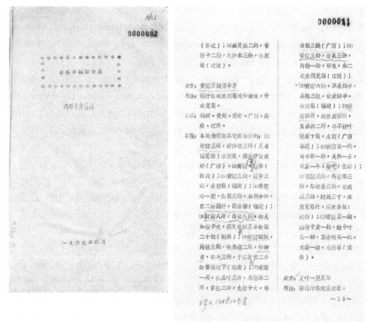

The front cover and contents page of the Collection of Secret Proven Prescriptions for Malaria, *April 1969*

She decided to start with historical research. She collected and sorted the medical writings from past dynasties, referred to prescriptions offered by the general public and consulted veteran doctors of TCM. In just three months, she had collected more than 2,000 prescriptions, including medicines for oral and external uses and those derived from plants, animals and minerals. On this basis, she compiled *A Collection of Secret Proven Prescriptions for*

Malaria, which contained 640 prescriptions. In April 1969, the book was sent to the '523' office and forwarded to related units for reference.

Artemisia annua, from which artemisinin would eventually be extracted, was included in these prescriptions.

However, artemisinin did not feature in Tu Youyou's initial round of medicine screenings and tests. The central task was to look for a suitable TCM to deal with vomiting, a side effect caused by dichroine, a type of alkaloid, through the compatibility of medicines. She combined some antiemetic TCMs with orixine and conducted pharmacological experiments on the vomiting models of pigeons and cats. However, even the best combination had no effect on cats, only on pigeons.

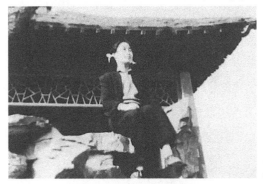

Tu Youyou in Hainan's Changjiang malaria area in 1969

In May 1969, she started preparing TCM water extracts and ethyl alcohol extracts and sending them to the Academy of Military Medical Sciences for anti-malaria screening. By the end of June, more than 50 samples had been sent. It was found that pepper extracts had an 84% suppression rate against malaria plasmodia in mice, which was an encouraging figure. However, the results of subsequent research were not as she expected. Tu Youyou found that, while pepper extracts could improve malaria symptoms, they were not successful in eradicating the disease.

In July 1969, members of the '523' project were sent to malaria areas in Hainan province. The '523' office required the Institute of Chinese Materia Medica to send three researchers there and proposed that the peppers, chilies and alums that showed a high inhibition ratio to mouse malaria in the sample screenings in the first half of the year should be taken for clinical curative effect observation.

The Institute of Chinese Materia Medica assigned Tu Youyou and two other researchers to Hainan. According to the clinical verifications of malaria in Hainan, although the inhibition ratio of the prepared samples of peppers, chilies and alums exceeded 80%, these samples could only improve the symptoms of malaria patients and couldn't prevent plasmodium from becoming active in the patient.After the project was finished, Tu Youyou was conferred the title 'Excellent Member' by the Guangdong '523' office.

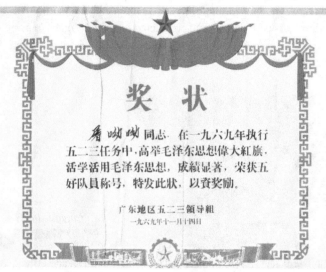

In 1969, Tu Youyou was given the title 'Excellent Member' while executing the '523' project

In 1970, the research group focused on further research into peppers. From February to September, more than 120 samples of extracts and compounds, including peppers, were sent for testing to the Academy of Military Medical Sciences. Experiments showed that the effectiveness of pepper could not be improved by separation and purification; although it could be enhanced by adjusting the proportion of ingredients, the effectiveness of pepper was much lower than that of chloroquine.

At the Guangzhou meeting in 1971, it was once again declared that the 523 project involving TCM research should continue rather than be suspended. Therefore, the research group led by Tu Youyou was expanded to four members, meaning that Tu now had three assistants.

By the beginning of September 1971, they had screened more than 200 samples of water and alcohol extracts from more than 100 TCMs. They expected to secure some significant findings, but the results were disappointing.

Among those screened TCMs, the highest inhibition ratio found against plasmodium was just 40%.

Could it be that the historical records were unreliable?

Could it be that there was something wrong with the experimental procedure?

Was it possible that nothing useful could be found in the treasure of TCM?

They hadn't found any new medicine more effective than chloroquine or antipyretic dichroa. Had they reached the end of the road?

The No. 191 Sample

"Let's immerse ourselves in reading the medical books again!" said Tu Youyou. Her stubborn perseverance inspired other people. From *Shennong's Herbal* to *The Complete Record of Holy Benevolence* and *Treatise on the Differentiation* and *Treatment of Epidemic Febrile Disease*, the pages of the medical books were curled at the edges through constant reading.

For a long time, Artemisia annua, commonly known as sweet wormwood and part of the asteraceae family, didn't receive much attention, until one day Tu Youyou decided to try extracting it using diethyl ether (instead of water or ethyl alcohol) at a boiling point of 34.6°C.

This method grasped the root of the matter – temperature was the key to the extraction of artemisinin.

With a history of more than 2,000 years in China, the usage of Artemisia annua as a medicine was first recorded in the silk book *Prescriptions of 52 Diseases*, which was excavated in tomb number three in the Han dynasty tombs in Mawangdui, Changsha, and also recorded in ancient books and records such as *Shennong's Herbal*. Artemisia annua had been first used to treat malaria in AD340 according to *A Handbook of Prescriptions for Emergencies* by Ge Hong of the Eastern Jin dynasty (317-420). Later, 'Artemisia annua decoction', 'Artemisia annua pills' and 'Artemisia annua powder to prevent malaria' were recorded in *The Complete Record of Holy Benevolence* of the Song dynasty (960-1276), *Danxi's Mastery of Medicine* of the Yuan dynasty (1206-1368) and *Prescriptions for Universal Relief* of the Ming dynasty (1368-1644), respectively. Li Shizhen of the Ming dynasty included the experience of his predecessors and cases of malaria treatment in the *Compendium of Materia Medica*. The application of Artemisia annua in malaria treatment was also recorded in the *Treatise on the Differentiation and Treatment of Epidemic Febrile Disease* and *Essentials of Materia Medica* of the Qin dynasty (1616-1912), and it was also popular in folk medicine.

During repeated study of the literature, Tu Youyou was enlightened by the words "Soak a handful of Artemisia annua in two liters of water; extract juice from the water and drink it down" in *A Handbook of Prescriptions for Emergencies.*

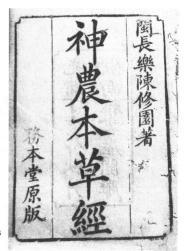

Artemisia annua is recorded in Shennong's Herbal, *the earliest TCM book*

This scene would be described in legend as follows: Reading *A Handbook of Prescriptions for Emergencies* by Ge Hong early in the morning or late at night, Tu Youyou was inspired by the ancient prescription: "Soak a handful of Artemisia annua in two liters of water; extract juice from the water and drink it down."

However, the actual experiment was difficult and complicated. In *Artemisia Annua and Artemisinin-Based Drugs* published in 2009, Tu referred to a series of experiments of that time.

As the book pointed out, the artemisinin monomer obtained after separation retains stable anti-malaria effects after being boiled for half an hour: "It can be inferred that the temperature rise will negatively influence the anti-malaria effects of artemisinin only when some substances coexist in crude drugs during crude extraction."

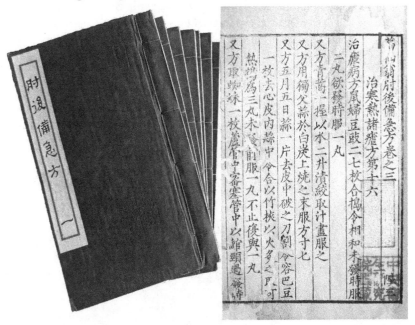

Artemisia annua had been used to treat malaria since AD340, according to **A Handbook of Prescriptions for Emergencies** *by Ge Hong of the Eastern Jin dynasty*

Why did the ancients perform 'juice extraction'? In previous extraction research, traditional Chinese herbal medicines were generally boiled in water or extracted with ethyl alcohol, but the results were unsatisfactory. Could it be that the effective constituents of Artemisi annua would be influenced by high temperature or enzymes? How could 'juice' be extracted from Artemisia annua? Since Artemisia annua could be extracted only from tender branches and leaves, does its extraction have something to do with the picking season and the parts of the plant used as herbal medicine?

After thorough consideration, Tu Youyou redesigned the research program. She also designed multiple plans for several key drugs. For example, Artemisia annua must be extracted at low temperatures and not above 60°C, and extraction was conducted with several solvents including water, ethyl alcohol and diethyl ether, and stalks and leaves were extracted separately.

The research group adopted the new program in September 1971 and screened and studied day and night key drugs that had been screened before, along with dozens of newly selected drugs.

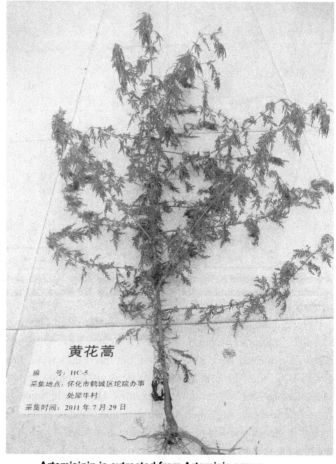

Artemisinin is extracted from Artemisia annua

After many sleepless nights, they proved that ether extracts of Artemisia annua had the best effects. Like the first light of morning, the team was buoyed once more after hundreds of failures.

The acidic extracts were highly toxic and ineffective, and the remaining neutral extracts were the effective constituents. After many sleepless nights, this pivotal finding made Tu Youyou feel excited.

Zhong Yurong, a member of the research group, lived in the research institute, which was two minute's walk away from the laboratory. After dinner, she would go back there to work with her colleagues until 9-10pm every evening.

In early October 1971, Tu Youyou was busy working with her research group. They were screening the samples strictly according to the procedure once again after 190 failures.

On October 4, all eyes nervously stared at the result of the No. 191 Artemisia annua ether neutral extract sample in the anti-malaria experiment.

The inhibition ratio against plasmodium reached 100%!

With the announcement of this test result, the whole laboratory became exulted.

The extracts were black and pasty. Though several processes still needed to be performed to obtain artemisinin crystals, it was clear that the key to success had been found.

Voluntary 'Guinea Pigs'

In order to further the clinical research, a large quantity of Artemisia annua extracts extracted with diethyl ether needed to be prepared for conducting preclinical toxicity tests and creating the drugs for clinical observation.

It is extremely difficult to obtain a large quantity of Artemisia annua extracts at short notice. The research work was at a standstill during the 'Cultural Revolution' and no pharmaceutical factories could cooperate with the research group. Tu Youyou's husband Li Tingzhao was very worried about his wife during that period in which she flung herself into her research. He said: "All she thought about was Artemisia annua. She returned home smelling of alcohol and suffered from toxic hepatitis."

Toxic hepatitis can be caused by organic solvents such as diethyl ether.

Zhong Yurong recalled that the research group adopted a folk recipe in which the conventional laboratory extraction vessels were replaced by the seven water storage vats to shorten research time. Then, more researchers were appointed by the Institute of Chinese Materia Medica to assist them with the extraction of Artemisia annua using diethyl ether.

"Organic solvents like diethyl ether are harmful to health," Jiang Tingliang said. "The facilities then were simple and crude. There were neither ventilation systems nor protective devices. Researchers just wore gauze masks."

Gradually, researchers felt dizzy and their eyes became swollen. They also exhibited other symptoms such as nosebleeds and skin allergies.

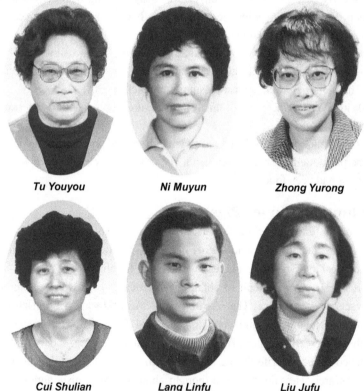

Tu Youyou *Ni Muyun* *Zhong Yurong*

Cui Shulian *Lang Linfu* *Liu Jufu*

Some important members of the research group involved in the discovery of artemisinin

Neutral extracts extracted with diethyl ether were available, but a problem arose during the preclinical test in that suspected toxic side effects were found in the pathological sections of certain animals. The problem remained unsolved after several animal tests. Was it caused by the animals or the drugs? The disputes among researchers in the laboratory were intense: the research group held that the problem was not serious since Artemisia annua was not highly toxic according to the ancient books and several animal tests that had been conducted; while the colleagues engaged in toxicology and pharmacology insisted that the clinical tests could be conducted only after the safety of extracts was confirmed.

"I was worried. Malaria is a seasonal infectious disease. I really didn't want to miss the clinical observation season, or else I would have to wait for another year," said Tu Youyou.

In order to apply Artemisia annua neutral extracts extracted with diethyl ether No. 191 in clinical experiments with immediate effect, Tu Youyou submitted a report to the leader based on a comprehensive analysis of the application of Artemisia annua in ancient times and the results of the animal tests.

"I'm group leader. It's my responsibility to try the medicine first!" she insisted. Her attitude surprised many; it was impressive that this gentle, bespectacled woman from south of the Yangtze river was so courageous.

"It was extremely difficult to conduct tests at that time. Scientists used themselves as 'human guinea pigs'; it showed their spirit of devotion," said Shi Yigong, vice-president of Tsinghua University.

"This spirit of devotion was particularly important," Jiang Tingliang recalled.

Tu Youyou's proposal to volunteer to try the medicine received a positive response from her colleagues in the research group. In July 1972, Tu Youyou and two other researchers were admitted to Beijing Dongzhimen hospital and became the first batch of 'guinea pigs' to try the medicine. They took it and received one-week observation under the close monitoring of the hospital. No significant toxic side effects of the extracts were found. In order to fully prove the safety of the middle trunk extracts extracted with diethyl ether, the research group conducted another five tests in which larger doses were taken by human subjects; it was demonstrated that the subjects remained in a healthy condition.

From August to October 1972, taking the extracts with her, Tu Youyou went to the malaria areas in Changjiang, Hainan province. Her group travelled over land and water in the hot weather, seizing every opportunity to find patients.

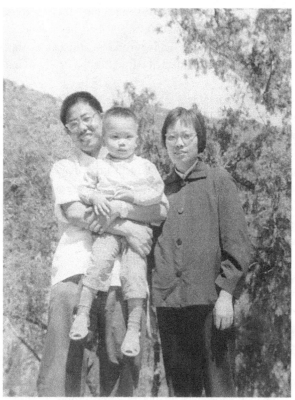

Zhong Yurong, her husband Yan Shuchang and their son. Yan Shuchang also worked in the Institute of Chinese Materia Medica. He actively responded to Tu Youyou's proposal and volunteered to take the medicine

In the first clinical experiment, carefulness and prudence were paramount and the dosage had to be increased gradually. Three dose groups were set by Tu Youyou according to her own medicine trial procedures. The selected patients included natives with high immunity and non-natives lacking immunity; the types of malaria ranged from vivax malaria to falciparum malaria. Tu Youyou personally administered the medicine to her patients to ensure the dose and stayed by their bedsides to observe their condition and take their temperature. She also carefully studied changes in the plasmodia count after blood smear tests.

Finally, Tu observed the clinical anti-malaria effects of 21 cases, comprising 11 cases of vivax malaria, nine cases of falciparum malaria and one case of mixed infection. The clinical outcome was satisfactory: the average fever abatement times for vivax malaria and falciparum malaria were 19 hours and 36 hours respectively. In all cases, the plasmodia became negative.

In the same year, another nine cases were tested in Beijing 302 hospital and satisfactory results were obtained.

The Discovery of Artemisinin

Tu Youyou's research efforts didn't let up despite her team's phased success. In no time, she and her colleagues started to purify and separate the effective components in Artemisia annua extracts extracted with diethl ether.

The sweet wormwood growing in Beijing contained only a very small quantity of artemisinin, which made it more difficult for researchers to discover. Moreover, the discovery of artemisinin was also compromised by the collecting season and the technology of purification.

From April 26 to June 26, 1972, the research group obtained small amounts of granular, sheet or needle-shaped crystals. Each time there was a new achievement in the separation and extraction, the laboratory broke into cheers and applause.

To obtain the effective anti-malaria monocrystal earlier, every member in the group strived to find the right solution.

When Tu Youyou went to Hainan to verify the clinical curative effect of middle trunk extracts extracted with diethyl ether, the practical work of the research group in Beijing was arranged by Ni Muyun. Then, the research group separated several crystals on September 25, September 29, October 25, October 30 and November 8, 1972, based on the purified samples of polyamide.

自1971年7月以来，我们筛选了中草药单、复方等一百多
种。发现青蒿（黄花蒿 Artemisia annua L. 係菊科植物。按中医认
为此药主治骨蒸烦热。但在唐、宋、元、明医籍、本草及民间都曾
提到有治疟作用的乙醇提取物对鼠疟模型有95%～100%的抑
制效价。以后进一步提取，去除其中无效而毒性又比较集中的酸性
部分。得到有效的中性部分。12月下旬。在鼠疟模型基础上，又
用乙醚提取物与中性部分分别进行了猴疟实验。结果与鼠疟相同。

~1~

通过多方面的分析。我们挑选一部分药物，进一步复筛。复筛
时参考民间用药经验。改进提取方法并增设多剂量组。探索药物剂
量与效价的关系。经过反复实践。终于使青蒿的动物效价。由30
～40%提高到95%以上。青蒿的水煎剂是无效的。95%乙醇
提取物的效价也不好。只有30～40%左右。后来从本草及民间
"绞汁"服用中得到启发。使我们考虑到有效成分可能在亲脂部分。
于是改用乙醚提取。这样动物效价才有了显著的提高。经过比较。
发现乙醇提取物虽然也含有乙醚提取的物质。但是杂质多了$\frac{2}{3}$左右。
这就大大影响了有效成分充分显示应有的效价。另外药物的采收季
节对效价也是有影响的。在这点上我们走过一点弯路。开始我们只
注意品种问题。了解到北京市售青蒿都是北京近郊产的黄花蒿，不

~5~

Part of the report submitted by the research group of malaria prevention and treatment of the Academy of TCM at the meeting held in Nanjing in 1972

No sooner had Tu Youyou returned to Beijing from the malaria areas of Hainan than she threw herself into chemical research. She discussed and analyzed the obtained chemical monomers with the research group. Similarities and differences were identified by chromogenic reaction, plate chromatography, Rf value and so on, separated constituents were integrated and the drug's effects on mouse malaria were evaluated.

At the beginning of December, the mouse malaria experiment found that the crystals obtained on November 8 by Zhong Yurong had obvious effects. The plasmodium became negative after the mouse was fed 50mg of the medicine per kilogram of its body weight. Thus, the research group declared November 8, 1972 to be the birthday of artemisinin.

This was the first time that a single compound obtained from Artemisia annua was proven to have anti-malaria medicinal effects.

When the news that artemisinin could be used as an anti-malaria drug was spread nationwide, the Institute of Chinese Materia Medica began receiving letters and visitors from various places shortly after New Year's Day 1973. Tu Youyou personally replied to letters, delivered materials and warmly received visitors, explaining Artemisia annua, Artemisia annua extracts and her team's chemical research progress in detail. Soon, many research groups in Yunnan, Shandong and elsewhere were referring to her methods in researching Artemisia annua.

Chapter 4

A Miracle Chinese Medicine

Unsatisfactory Result in the First Clinical Observation

After modifying and improving the procedure of large-scale extraction in the laboratory, Tu Youyou and her colleagues started a new round of hard work. Though the lab conditions were poor, the research group made the best of them. Some 100g of pure artemisinin had been obtained between January and May 1973, and Tu divided it into four parts: one part for chemical research, one for preclinical safety tests, another for the preparation of drugs for clinical observation and a small quantity for reserve.

Artemisinin safety tests on cats were conducted in the second quarter of 1973, when it was shown to have no obvious influence on blood pressure, heart rate or heart rhythm, regardless of the size of dose. In three batches of toxicity tests on dogs, the indicators were normal except in some cases where dogs salivated, vomited or had diarrhea; no obvious toxic side-effects were found.

As a precaution, tests were also conducted on healthy human subjects. After a detailed plan for human trials, four researchers took the medicine between July 21 and August 10, 1973, and again no obvious toxic side-effects were found.

With the animal and human safety tests for artemisinin completed, a new anti-malaria drug was about to be born. Everyone looked forward to clinical verification; however, the process was full of twists and turns.

Colleagues from the Institute of Materia Medica sent artemisinin tablets to Hainan and doctors from the Institute of Acupuncture and Moxibustion and the CACMS were responsible for clinical observation.

Eight malaria cases of non-Hainan natives were treated with artemisinin from August 10 to October 15, 1973, and the trials were conducted in two stages.

The treatment effects of artemisinin in five falciparum malaria cases of non-natives were observed before September 22. It was shown to be effective in only one case; the amount of plasmodia in two cases was reduced but the patients stopped taking the medicine before the end of the trial due to contractions of their heart beats; and it was ineffective in the other two cases. The results were unsatisfactory.

Unsatisfactory results had been obtained in the first clinical observation of artemisinin!

The news was sent to Beijing by phone, and everyone was shocked. Tu Youyou and her group were beset with numerous questions. They set out to find the answers. The purity of the artemisinin was standard and the data of the animal tests was reliable. Could it be that something had been wrong with the form of the drug? They asked their colleagues who were conducting the clinical tests in Hainan to send the tablets to Beijing. On examination, they found that the remaining tablets were very hard; they couldn't be crushed in a pestle and mortar. They knew then that the problem lay in disintegration, which had influenced absorption of the drug.

Tu's research group decided to put raw artemisinin powder in capsules and complete clinical verification before the season for field observation in the malaria endemic area in Hainan ended, so as to determine whether it had clinical effects.

Tu Youyou capsulized the artemisinin herself. Zhang Guozhen, the deputy director of the Institute of Chinese Materia Medica, undertook the arduous task of transporting the capsules to Hainan. He arrived in the epidemic area on September 29. Three vivax malaria cases of non-natives were observed and each took 3-3.5g of the medicine. The results showed that, after taking the medicine, the patients' temperatures became normal within an average of 31 hours, and the plasmodium became negative within 18-and-a-half hours. Artemisinin was effective in all cases, with no obvious side effects. Clinical verification was stopped because the season for field observation in the malaria endemic area of Hainan was over. This was the first clinical trial of artemisinin. It proved that the artemisinin obtained by

Tu's research group was the effective anti-malaria constituent of Artemisia annua.

Colleagues from the Institute of Acupuncture and the Moxibustion China Academy of Chinese Medical Science wrote a report on the results of the first clinical observation of artemisinin and submitted it to the '523' office. The report failed to state that two different dosage forms were used in the eight cases and that observations of the eight cases were completed in two stages. That is why the report was later misinterpreted by some people; it was simply a misunderstanding.

Setbacks were interwoven with success in the first clinical verification of artemisinin. The three cases using artemisinin capsules indicated that the clinical and laboratory effects of artemisinin were the same.

A new anti-malaria medicine was born!

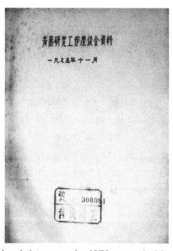

Observation of the effects of artemisinin II in eight cases in 1973 recorded in the document Materials of Symposium Artemisia Annua Research (November 1975), *kept at the Shanghai Institute of Organic Chemistry*

According to the records, the research group determined in April 1973 that artemisinin was a non-nitrogenous compound. Artemisinin had a molecular weight of 282 and its molecular formula was $C_{15}H_{22}O_5$; it belonged to sesquiterpenoids.[1] It indicated that artemisinin was the effective constituent in the clinical verification undertaken in Hainan in the second half of 1973.

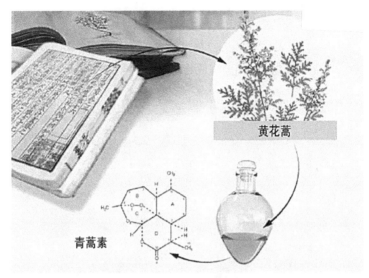

The discovery process of artemisinin

A meeting on medical research for malaria prevention and treatment (chemical synthesis) was held in Shangqiu, Henan province in April 1974. Chen Mei from the science and education department was appointed by the Institute of Chinese Materia Medica to attend the meeting. He took the artemisinin research materials and gave a report on the research progress of artemisinin and dihydroartemisinin. It was the first time that artemisinin had been discussed in an internal professional meeting.

The Institute of Chinese Materia Medica studied its structure in cooperation with the Shanghai Institute of Organic Chemistry, and did so using the X-ray diffraction method in cooperation with the Institute of Biophysics of the CAS. At the end of 1975, the three-dimensional structure of artemisinin was confirmed using the X-ray diffraction method. The structure of artemisinin was published for the first time in 1977.

Later, as requested by the Institute of Chinese Materia Medica in February 1976 and February 1977, the Ministry of Health approved the paper to be published in the *Chinese Science Bulletin* under the title 'Artemisinin Structure Coordinating Research Group'. Following that, Tu Youyou's research group introduced artemisinin in journals including *Plant Medica, Acta Pharmaceutica Sinica* and *Nature Medicine.*

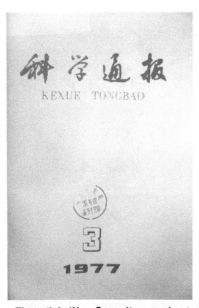

The article 'New Sesquiterpene Lactone-Artemisinin' was published in Chinese Science Bulletin *under the title the Artemisinin Structure Coordinating Research Group in 1977*

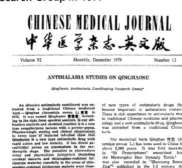

A paper published by Tu Youyou's research group

A Miracle Chinese Medicine

Planta
Journal of Medicinal Plant Research **medica**

Hippokrates

ISSN 0032-0943
Hippokrates Verlag Stuttgart

1982, Vol. 44, pp. 143–145. © Hippokrates Verlag GmbH

Journal of Medicinal Plant Research **medica**

Studies on the Constituents of Artemisia annua Part II[1]

Tu You-you, Ni Mu-yun, Zhong Yu-rong, Li Lan-na, Cui Shu-lian, Zhang Mu-qun, Wang Xiu-zhen, Ji Zheng[*] and Liang Xiao-tian[*]

[*] Institute of Chinese Materia Medica, Academy of Traditional Chinese Medicine, Beijing, China

Key Word Index:

Artemisia annua L.; Compositae; Qinghaosu; Qinghaosu I–V; Qinghao acid; Flavones, Alkanol; Scopoletin; Essential oil.

Abstract

The present paper is a continuation of our study on the Chinese traditional herb Artemisia annua L. [1–5], describing several additional constituents: qinghaosu IV and V (VII), qinghao acid (VIII) [6], chrysosplenol (VIa) [7] and a paraffinic alcohol. V, VII and VIII are compounds with unreported structures.

Introduction

A number of our earlier papers have been devoted to studies of chemical constituents isolated from Artemisia annua L. (Compositae), the most notable constituent being the antimalarial qinghaosu (I) [1–4], a peroxidic lactone with unique structure. Other constituents include qinghaosu I–III (II–IV), a flavonol (VI), scopoletin and a few terpenes from the essential oil [5].

This paper deals with the isolation and characterization of V, VIa, VII, VIII and a paraffinic alcohol. It is pertinent here to point out the close stereochemical kinship among the previously established structures I–IV. They all belong to the amorphane series (IX) [8], which has a cis-decalin skeleton with the isopropyl group trans to the hydrogen on the ring juncture. Compounds I and IV are further distinguished by the presence of a modified seven-membered A-ring as the result of insertion of an extra ether oxygen.

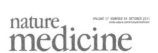

---

nature medicine

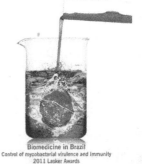

Biomedicine in Brazil
Control of mycobacterial virulence and immunity
2011 Lasker Awards

LASKER~DEBAKEY CLINICAL MEDICAL RESEARCH AWARD

COMMENTARY

The discovery of artemisinin (qinghaosu) and gifts from Chinese medicine

Youyou Tu

A paper by Tu Youyou and her research group introducing the chemical component and discovery of artemisinin published in Planta Medica *and* Nature Medicine

The Birth of 'Cotecxin'

In 1995, in the severely malaria-afflicted area of Kisumu, in Kenya, a mother contracted malaria during pregnancy. If she had taken traditional quinine or chloroquine for treatment, she might have survived, but her child might have been aborted or born with abnormalities. After using the Chinese artemisinin anti-malarial medicine 'Cotecxin' for treatment, the mother amazingly not only survived but also gave birth to a healthy baby! She kissed her baby again and again and named her Cotecxin to remind her of the life-saving grace of this Chinese medicine.

The birth of Cotecxin was derived from artemisinin derivative experiments carried out by Tu Youyou in late September 1973.

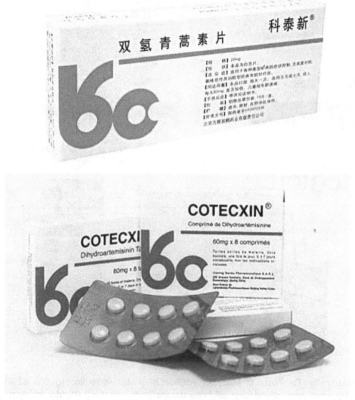

Cotecxin, one type of artemisinin anti-malaria medicine sold across the world

The discovery of artemisinin drew great attention from members of the Institute of Chinese Materia Medica of the China Academy of Chinese Medical Sciences, who offered great support in terms of manpower and material resources such as instruments and laboratories. Tu Youyou was responsible for the overall work. While organizing researchers to extract a large quantity of artemisinin and preparing clinical research, she changed her work focus to chemical research into artemisinin.

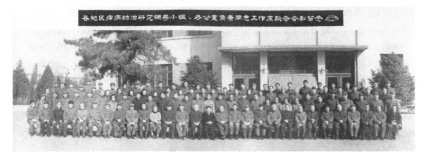

Group photo taken in 1977 of those in charge of 'Mission 523' from various regions. Tu Youyou is seventh from left in the second row

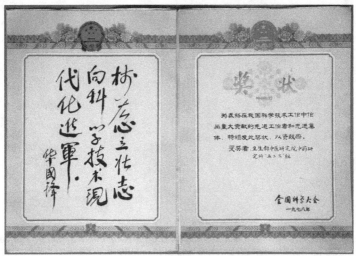

At the national conference on science and technology in 1978, the 'Mission 523' group of the Institute of Chinese Materia Medica, the China Academy of Chinese Medical Sciences and the Ministry of Health won the national advanced worker and advanced collective awards

In late September 1973, Tu Youyou discovered in her artemisinin derivatives experiments that, after artemisinin was reduced with sodium borohydride, the carbonyl band disappeared. The result proved the existence of carbonyl in artemisinin and therefore hydroxyl was introduced into the structure of artemisinin. When this experiment was repeated by her colleagues in the research group, the results were the same. The molecular formula of this reduced derivative is $C_{15}H_{24}O_5$ and its molecular weight is 284. Its name is dihydroartemisinin (once known as 'reduced artemisinin'). Ni Muyun from the research group introduced acetyl when reducing the derivatives and this acetylate was more effective against rodent malaria, which meant that more derivatives could be produced after the introduction of hydroxyl in the artemisinin molecule, thereby creating the necessary conditions for research into the quantitative structure-activity relationship (QSAR) of artemisinin derivatives.

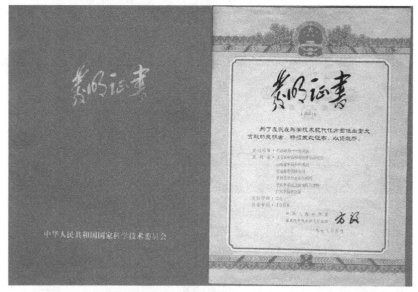

In September 1979, the new anti-malarial drug artemisinin won second prize at the national conference on science and technology

In 1975, the research group researched the QSAR of artemisinin, removal of the peroxide group and reduction of the laconic ring's carbonyl andacetylation. It was proved that the peroxide group in the structure of artemisinin was the active anti-malarial group under the premise of maintaining the peroxide group when the laconic ring's carbonyl was reduced into hydroxyl (i.e. dihydroartemisinin), which had a significant synergistic action. Its efficacy could be further increased by adding a certain side chain to the hydroxyl, and modifying the partial structure of artemisinin could change its physical and chemical properties and increase its anti-malarial activity. The relevant research information was reported to the '523' office. Dihydroartemisinin has a stronger anti-malarial effect than artemisinin, and it was also the precursor of synthesizing artemisinin-based drugs; other artemisinin-based anti-malarial drugs such as artesunate and artemether are based on dihydroartemisinin. Therefore, the discovery of dihydroartemisinin stood as another important contribution of Tu Youyou and her research group.

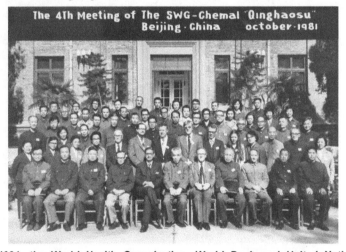

In 1981, the World Health Organization, World Bank and United Nations Development Program jointly held the fourth meeting of the scientific working group on the chemotherapy of malaria in Beijing, where a series of reports on artemisinin and its clinical application generated an enthusiastic response. This was an international academic exchange in which artemisinin succeeded in drawing global attention. Tu Youyou (fourth from left in the second row) made a speech at the meeting entitled 'Chemical Research on Artemisinin', which was subsequently published in the Journal of TCM

In October 1981, at an international meeting held in Beijing, a speech made by Tu Youyou entitled 'Chemical Research on Artemisinin' aroused great interest among experts from the World Health Organization (WHO), who considered that "the greater significance of this new discovery is to point out the direction for further designing and synthesizing new drugs".

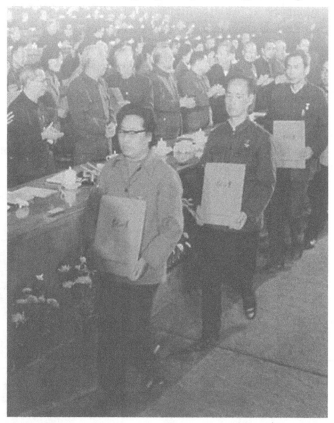

In October 1982, Tu Youyou (closest to the camera), as the primary inventor of the first unit to discover artemisinin and the unit's sole representative at the conference, accepted a certificate and badge of invention at the national awards conference for science and technology

The research results of the structure-function relationship spurred Tu Youyou to ponder further and she came to the firm belief that dihydroartemisinin was extremely worthy of further research and development. Fighting off objections, and shortly before completing the application for a new drug certificate for artemisinin in 1985, Tu led a new research program into pharmacy-related dihydroartemisinin and arranged for Fu Hangyu to be responsible for experimental research into pharmacology and other fields. They organized cooperative units to start research and development work on the new anti-malarial drug dihydroartemisinin and dihydroartemisinin tablets according to the requirements of the *Measures for the Examination and Approval of New Pharmaceuticals*. After seven years of hard work, they finally obtained the new drug certificate in 1992 for the discovery of dihydroartemisinin in 1973, and licensed it for production. This was another important contribution of Tu Youyou to the people of China and the world. The research into 'dihydroartemisinin and dihydroartemisinin tablets' that she led in those years was rated among the top 10 national scientific and technological achievements of the year, and she was subsequently employed by the CACMS as a tenured researcher.

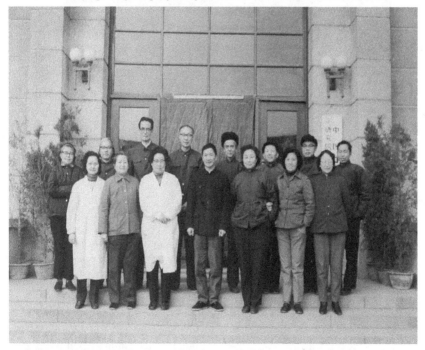

Colleagues from the Institute of Chinese Materia Medica of the Academy of TCM in 1985. Tu Youyou is third from left in the front row; fourth from the left is Jiang Tingliang, director of the institute

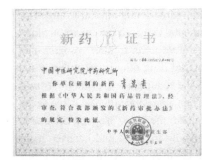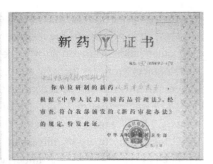

Left: New drug certificate of artemisinin issued by the Ministry of Health on October 3, 1986

Right: New drug certificate of dihydroartemisinin tablets issued by the Ministry of Health on July 20, 1992

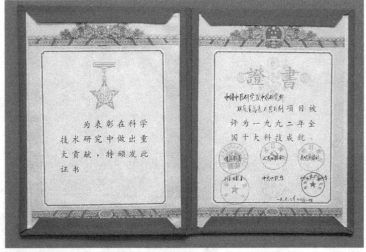

In December 1992, 'dihydroartemisinin and dihydroartemisinin tablets' were rated as one of the top 10 national scientific and technological achievements

As the clinical efficacy of dihydroartemisinin increased 10-fold, its dosage was reduced and its recrudescence rate was lowered to 1.95%, which further demonstrated the 'high efficacy, fast-acting and low toxicity' characteristics of artemisinin-based medicines. The name of that African girl, Cotecxin, was the name given to dihydroartemisinin after it was put into production by a pharmaceutical enterprise and widely used for the treatment of various types of malaria. For a very long period of time,

Cotecxin was even a standard gift given by Chinese leade
Africa, and it was honored as a 'magical Chinese medicine
continent.

According to statistics from the WHO, there are more than 2bn people living in areas with a high prevalence of malaria, including parts of Africa, Southeast Asia, South Asia and South America. Since 2000, about 240m people in Sub-Saharan Africa have benefited from artemisinin-based combination therapies (ACTs), and it has helped save the lives of about 1.5m people infected with malaria.

To further improve its efficacy, Chinese scientists have also developed artesunate, artemether and other new drugs. Of these, the artesunate injection has completely replaced the quinine injection and is highly recommended by the WHO for the treatment of severe malaria. It has saved the lives of more than 7m severe malaria patients (mainly children under five) in more than 30 countries across the world.

This ancient 'Chinese herb' is delivering a power that amazes the world.

Nationwide Cooperation Creates a Miracle

In 2011, Tu Youyou won the Lasker award (now known as the Lasker-Debakey Clinical Medical Research award), and regarded as 'the Nobel prize in the medical field' because of three 'firsts': the first person to bring artemisinin to the 'Mission 523' program group, the first person to extract artemisinin with an inhibition rate of 100% and the first to carry out clinical trials.

Her family and friends were delighted by this award, while Tu Youyou herself remained quite calm and repeatedly emphasized: "This is an honor not only for me but for all Chinese scientists."

'Miracle created by nationwide cooperation' is not a cliché, but a fact proven repeatedly during the research and development of artemisinin. The research process of artemisinin was not only full of the painstaking efforts of Tu Youyou and her research team, but also relied on nationwide collaboration and support.

The *Artemisinin Expertise Report* recorded that, since 1972, 10 provinces, regions and cities across the country had carried out clinical trials on 6,555 cases with Artemisia annua products and artemisinin products. These places included Hainan, Yunnan, Sichuan, Shandong,

Henan, Jiangsu, Hubei, southeast Asia and other areas where falciparum malaria and vivax malaria were prevalent, and 2,099 cases were treated with artemisinin products.

The research and development of the drugs was a long process that went from topic selection and project approval to the determination of technical route, from medicinal materials selection to compound extraction, and from pharmacology and toxicology to clinical trials. For such enormous and systematic work, multifarious cooperation would still be necessary even today.

Since 2010, Louis Miller, academician at the US National Academy of Sciences, had been engaged in recommending Tu Youyou and her artemisinin achievements to the relevant committees of the Lasker award and the Nobel prize.

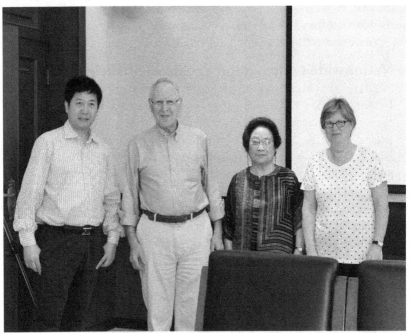

On June 19, 2013, Professor Louis Miller (second from left), academician at the US National Academy of Sciences, visited the Institute of Chinese Materia Medica of the CACMS. Second from right is Tu Youyou and far left is Chen Shilin, director of the Institute of Chinese Materia Medica

A Miracle Chinese Medicine

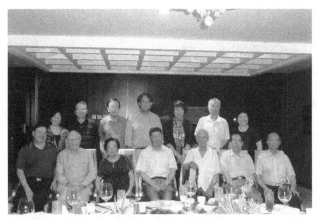

Professor Louis Miller with leading members of 'Mission 523': Tu Youyou (third from left in the front row); Zhang Jianfang (third from right in the front row); Li Guoqiao (far right in the front row); Luo Zeyuan (far right in the second row); Shi Linrong (second from right in the second row)

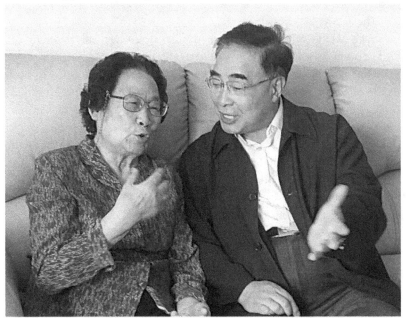

Zhang Boli, academician of the Chinese Academy of Engineering and president of the CACMS, talks with Tu Youyou about the extended research of artemisinin

Academician Zhang Boli, president of the CACMS, said: "The research on artemisinin was a long journey in which hundreds of scientists from dozens of scientific research units explored together. The nationwide cooperation system played an extremely important role in the research that was carried out under difficult conditions, and such a spirit of teamwork will never become outdated!"

The research process and results indicated that the 'Mission 523' search for anti-malarial drugs was a scientific research project involving nationwide scientific and technological cooperation in the years of the 'Cultural Revolution', a special historical period. In 1967, this project was launched and involved more than 500 scientific researchers from more than 60 scientific research units. On November 28, 1978, more than 100 people from six major research units and 39 major cooperative units attended an artemisinin appraisal meeting in Yangzhou.

Was it really necessary for so many units and people to research a new drug?

The answer is definitely yes.

Take the identification process of the stereochemical structure of artemisinin as an example. More than 40 years ago, as a state-level organization, the Institute of Chinese Materia Medica of the CACMS was short of advanced instruments and equipment, while the Shanghai Institute of Organic Chemistry could offer the best conditions for chemical research in China. Therefore, the two institutes cooperated for more than two years on researching the chemical construction of artemisinin, but without success. Then the Institute of Biophysics of the CAS joined the research and finally succeeded in identifying its structure by using advanced X-ray crystallography.

As the organizer and coordinator of this collaboration, the head office of 'Mission 523' offered great support in the discovery of artemisinin. When the Institute of Chinese Materia Medica found that the neutral ether extracts of Artemisia annua extracted with diethyl ether had a 100% inhibition rate against plasmodia in the mouse and simian malaria models, it instructed that clinical trials should be carried out that year; and when the institute obtained the artemisinin monomer, it again instructed that clinical trials should be conducted as soon as possible. At a symposium held for directors of the local offices of 'Mission 523' from January 10 to 17, 1974, it was stated: "The CACMS would be in charge of coordinating the next research by organizing communication about the research of sweet wormwood among institutions in Yunnan, Shandong and other regions."

On February 5, 1974, the national leading team for the research of malaria control forwarded the brief report from the symposium held for directors of the local offices of 'Mission 523'. The brief report recommended the exchange of experiences in the research of antimalarial artemisinin. Based on the report, the CACMS held an artemisinin research symposium from February 28 to March 1, 1974. The participants comprised researchers from the Shandong Institute of TCM, the Shandong Institute of Parasitic Control, the Yunnan Institute of Materia Medica and the Beijing Institute of Materia Medica. At the symposium, they exchanged details on the progress of their three-year artemisinin research and made a division for future work in order to strengthen their collaboration, avoid overlap, coordinate tasks and accelerate the work. The Institute of Chinese Materia Medica invited the representatives to visit its artemisinin research laboratories, and offered them introductions to the symposium's participants. Nationwide collaboration had begun.

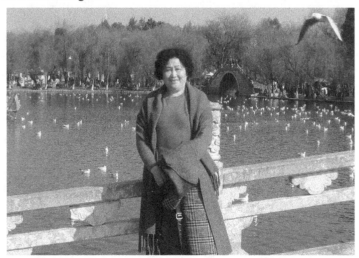

Luo Zeyuan, a researcher from the Yunnan Institute of Materia Medica, made outstanding contributions to artemisinin research

One year later, units from eight provinces and cities attended the Chengdu meeting and planed the 'great campaign' of Artemisia annua research, which led to a climax in the nationwide collaboration.

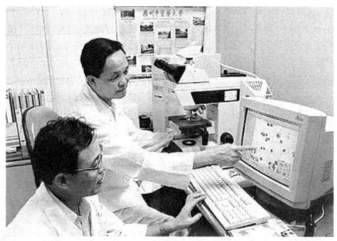

Li Guoqiao (right), chief professor of the Guangzhou University of Chinese Medicine, made significant contributions to clinical research into artemisinin

Zhang Jianfang, former vice-director of the National Leading Group Office for 'Mission 523', said: "The success in the research and development of artemisinin is a collective honor for all the researchers involved in China. The six research units made their own contributions. It was impossible for any one of the six units on the invention certificate to independently develop a drug with a new structure based on traditional medicine with modern technology, as talent, equipment, funds, theories and technologies were rather limited at that time."

Zhou Weishan, academician of the CAS, participated in 'Mission 523'. "The research and development of artemisinin drugs was a complex, systematic project involving numerous researchers," he sighed with emotion. "No single unit or individual could independently accomplish that research."

Field work in hyper-endemic areas of malaria was an important part of 'Mission 523', and it mainly comprised epidemiological investigation, the treatment of critical cases and clinical observation of medicine. Most hyper-endemic areas of malaria were in places with difficult natural environments and living conditions. The researchers needed to work hard and overcome difficulties over a period of months when carrying out the tasks in those areas. For example, a 40-strong working team was sent to Hainan island from Shanghai at the end of the 1960s. They had to trek over mountains and wade across rivers during their work. They overcame various difficulties such as tough living conditions, mountain-climbing and a fear of snakes. One example serves to demonstrate the living conditions. A team member once lodged with a local peasant. One day, he found a small frog in his bowl. After an intense 'mental struggle', he ate the frog in order to show his friendship towards the peasant under the difficult political conditions of that time. It's hard to imagine such field work being conducted today.

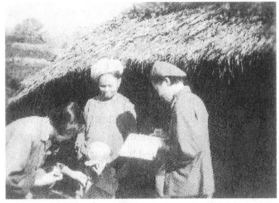

Researchers observe the effects of the new anti-malaria medicine in Yunnan province

The 'spirit of dedication' was emphasized in the scientific research of that time, and it could be found in all the research groups. According to the plan of 'Mission 523', research into the feeding and breeding of the Anopheles lesteri mosquito was assigned to the research institutions in Shanghai. International scientific research into the mating and breeding habits of anopheles mosquitoes needed strict conditions, including, for example, an oval feeding room at constant temperature and humidity. However, the research conditions in China were far from ideal at that time. Researchers worked in small and sweltering breeding rooms where mosquitoes would frequently bite their hands over a long period of time. When Shanghai No. 2 Pharmaceutical Factory needed to carry out simulative observations to develop a smell repellent, 26 PLA soldiers volunteered to be the subjects.

In order to verify its effectiveness, the mosquito-repellent was first applied to their ankles and gun belts; the soldiers then lay on the banks of a river where mosquitoes swarmed at night, and then counted how many times they were bitten by mosquitoes.

Another important feature of 'Mission 523' was collaboration. Research groups in the same field from different regions communicated with each other on a frequent and timely basis. For example, with regard to 'the leading research group of malaria immunity' in Shanghai, other research groups from different parts of China exchanged plans, summaries and brief reports. They also advised each other on their work and collaborated with a clear-cut division of labor. Before long, they wrote up their research on malaria immunity and distributed it between themselves. Their collaboration was fully affirmed by the national leading team of 'Mission 523', and it was promoted across the nation. In the special research system of 'Mission 523', many results were provided complete and promptly to its peers nationwide for reference.

The scientific research conditions were rather difficult in the 1960s and 1970s. Many researchers didn't put their names to their academic papers against a background of great nationwide collaboration. Their perseverance and enthusiasm for scientific research originated from a simple idea: it was what the country needed.

Those people, some of whose names were known while others were unknown, were like grass that was neither as fragrant as flowers, nor as tall as trees. However, their contributions would be engraved in history.

Artemisinin Saving the World

Malaria, along with Aids and cancer, is one of the world's principal life-threatening diseases listed by the WHO.

Before artemisinin was discovered and used extensively, nearly 400m people had become infected with malaria and at least 1m were dying of it every year. The infected and the dead were mainly concentrated in sub-Saharan Africa. Many people died simply because they couldn't afford expensive traditional anti-malaria medicine.

Therefore artemisinin has, without doubt, become a lifesaving medicine for those infected with malaria.

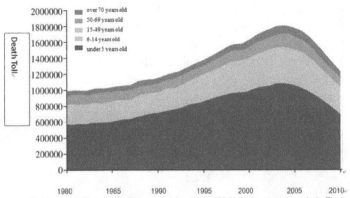

Data source: Christopher J L Murray et al. Global malaria mortality 1980-2010: A systematic analysis, The Lancet 2012, 379: 413-431.

Global malaria mortality between 1980 and 2010

As for the professionals, another value of artemisinin lies in its effectiveness in curing the malaria caused by anti-chloroquine plasmodium as well as overcoming multidrug-resistant strains of malaria. Artemisinin has demonstrated incredibly high cure rates for decades and it has been the most effective anti-malarial drug.

What is even more miraculous is that artemisinin burst onto the scene at a time when malaria patients had no effective drugs due to the rapid spread of chloroquine-resistant plasmodium.

Theoretically, the misuse of any medicine during its long-term application process could lead to lower sensibility and higher resistance, and even loss of efficacy. Therefore, the WHO emphasized that the use of malaria monotherapy must be banned and instead it recommended artemisinin-combination therapies. ACTs recommended by the WHO are a type of compound anti-malaria medicine that consists of quick-acting anti-malarial drugs such as dihydroartemisinin, artesunate and artemether, and long-acting anti-malarials such as piperaquine mefloquine and benflumetol.

Why don't plasmodiums easily develop resistance to artemisinin? The answer lies in its specific chemical bond known as the endoperoxide bridge, in the molecular structure of artemisinin, which is the key to killing plasmodium.

Due to the rapid effect of artemisinin, plasmodia don't have time to induce compositions of antioxidase and antioxidants. At the same time, red blood cells do not contain nuclei, so there are no chromosomes or genomes in red blood cells. It's impossible for red cells to enhance the expression of antioxidase genes. Therefore, lacking sufficient protection from antioxidant components, red blood cells as well as plasmodia parasitizing in them are scarcely capable of resisting fierce attacks from artemisinin. Once they encounter it, they are killed at once.

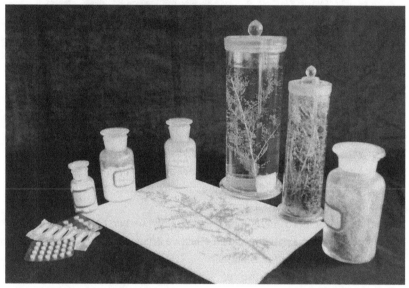

From right to left: herbarium of Artemisia apiacea, artemisinin and artemisinin tablets

Nowadays, ACTs are the standard treatment recommended by the WHO in the fight against malaria. The WHO believes that ACTs are the most effective drugs in curing malaria and in reducing resistance to anti-malarial medicine. As the discoverer and biggest producer of artemisinin, China has played a significant role in treating malaria all over the world.

In malarious areas of Africa, artemisinin has saved millions of lives. According to the statistics from the WHO, since 2000 nearly 240m people have benefited from ACTs, and nearly 1.5m have been completely cured in sub-Saharan Africa alone.

Mbery Kunath, the leader of anti-malaria projects in Zimbabwe's Ministry of Public Health, said that a tracking survey by the ministry between 2010 and 2013 showed that 97% of malaria patients who took artemisinin-based anti-malarial drugs had been cured. Artemisinin-based combination drugs have been used since 2008 in Zimbabwe. The country's malaria prevalence rate dropped from 15% in the early years of this century to 2.2% in 2013 because of the popularization of artemisinin-based anti-malarial drugs.

In KwaZulu-Natal, South Africa, compound artemether from China has reduced the number of malaria patients by 78% and deaths by 88%. And in Benin, west Africa, local people named the effective and cheap medicine given by Chinese medical teams "the wonder drug from the distant east"...

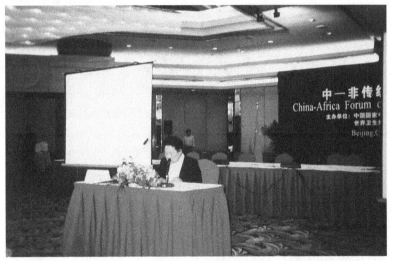

In October 2002, Tu Youyou was invited to the China-Africa Forum of Traditional Medicine Development and Cooperation, which was jointly held by China and the WHO. She produced a report entitled **Artemisinin: An Important Fruit of Traditional Anti-malarial Treatment**

Dr Matshidiso Rebecca Moeti, Regional Director for the WHO's Africa region, said that the discovery of artemisinin had contributed greatly to people's health across the world. "In Africa, many people, particularly children, are killed by malaria. It is the biggest health threat. For many years, artemisinin has saved many African lives, and it has played an important role for Africa to achieve its UN Millennium Development Goals."

Bernice Dahn, Liberia's Minister of Public Health, said: "Malaria is the biggest threat to people's health in my country." Previously, the Liberian government always used quinine and other treatments to tackle malaria but they had obvious side effects. Such worries were eliminated once they switched to artemisinin. "We appreciate the considerable medical assistance given to us by the Chinese government in conducting research into malaria control."

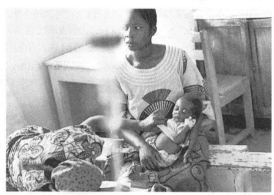

In Africa, a mother sits on a hospital bed, holding her malaria-affected child

Awa Marie Coll Seck, Senegal's Minister of Health, said that she herself had taken care of malaria patients over a number of years as a frontline medical worker so she knew that artemisinin worked effectively, and how it had brought hope to all malaria-affected countries in Africa.

"Malaria outbreaks occur every year in my country", said Alzouma Dari, deputy health minister of Niger. "I am very grateful for China's long-term medical assistance. We also use artemisinin medicine to control malaria, and it has achieved remarkable results."

Gabon's vice-minister of health, Célestine Ba Oguewa, said that China has made a great contribution to public health, and artemisinin has played an important role in malaria treatment, especially in those countries and regions with limited sanitary conditions.

Since the 1960s, the Chinese government has been dispatching medical teams to Africa to offer medical assistance in disease control. Until the end of 2009, it had funded the construction of 54 hospitals in Africa, established 30 centers for malaria control and prevention, and provided 35 African countries with anti-malarial medicines worth about Rmb200m.

On October 23, 2015, Bibi Ameenah Firdaus Gurib-Fakim, president of Mauritius, paid a visit to the Institute of Chinese Materia Medica of the CACMS during a visit to China. This president, also a famous biologist, congratulated Tu Youyou on receiving the Nobel prize. She said that Tu's work had made the whole world focus on traditional medicine again, which was not only important to China but also meaningful for developing countries and traditional medicine across the globe. With a keen interest on TCM, she said that Africa was also rich in traditional medicine and hoped to cooperate with China in traditional medicine so as to extend the platform of South-South cooperation. Mauritius would be the window leading TCM to the world.

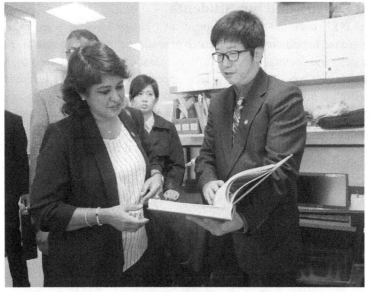

Bibi Ameenah Firdaus Gurib-Fakim, president of Mauritius, visits the Institute of TCM of the CACMS. Chen Shilin, director of the institute, shows her their research achievements, including artemisinin

Chapter 5

Worldwide Reputation

Tu Youyou and her Students

In 1981, once the China Academy of Chinese Medical Sciences was selected to be among the first batch of academic institutions able to grant master's and doctoral degrees, Tu Youyou started to enroll master's degree candidates. Over time, four students under her guidance were awarded a master's degree. Two of these students, Wu Chongming and Gu Yucheng, conducted research into the active ingredients or effective chemical components of TCMs such as Corydalis yanhusuo, Artemisia japonica, Cirsium japonicum and Cirsium setosum, and they adopted Tu Youyou's methods of researching artemisinin.

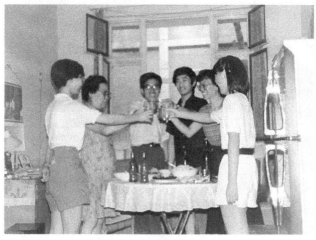

Tu Youyou invites colleagues and the postgraduate student Gu Yucheng (third from left) to her house, July 1987

After the Institute of Chinese Materia Medica was granted the authority to launch a PhD program in 2001, she recruited her doctoral student Wang Manyuan in 2002.

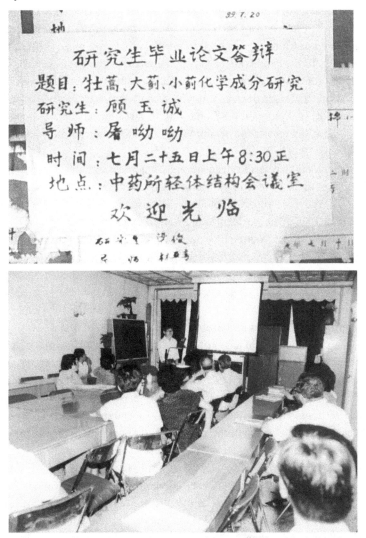

Tu Youyou's postgraduate student Gu Yucheng defends his graduate thesis, July 25, 1989

Combining the twin aims of training students and maintaining the integrity of her training plan, Tu Youyou guided Wang Manyuan in completing his PhD thesis on the preliminary study on chemical components and bioactivity of Chirita longgangensis var. hongyao. Hongyao, the whole plant of Chirita longgangensis W. T. Wang var. hongyao S. Z. Huang, is only found in China. It was used as a folk herbal drug in southern China, especially in the southwest of Guangxi Zhuang autonomous region. It is often used for the treatment of irregular menstruation, bodily weakness, anemia and traumatic fracture. Guiding Wang Yuanli took up a considerable amount of Tu Youyou's time and was in addition to her research into artemisinin, demonstrating her commitment to helping educate others even at the age of over 70.

Wang Manyuan is the dean of the Chinese pharmacy department of the school of TCM of Capital Medical University. He initially 'knew' his tutor Tu Youyou through a notebook. In this small, dark green notebook Tu Youyou recorded the detailed analysis of experiments and properties of TCM when, in her youth, she extracted and separated the materials used for TCM.

Tu Youyou gave the notebook to Wang Manyuan when he had just entered school in 2002. She hoped that it would help him learn more about phytochemistry. For Wang, the notebook, which recorded the chemical properties of TCM, was still useful and by no means out of date.

Wang said that the old pages of the notebook reminded him of a rigorous and senior scientist working at her desk every day. This notebook with 'Learning from comrade Lei Feng' (a selfless soldier in the People's Liberation Army) inscribed on the title page was completed during the late 1960s and early 1970s. At that time, Tu Youyou had just taken over 'Mission 523', tasked with the research and development of anti-malaria drugs. It was difficult to source scientific research materials then because much of the information on TCM could only be obtained from materials that were stored in the revolutionary committees of schools around China. Therefore, once Tu acquired scientific research materials, she would note down every single relevant detail in her notebook. Within three months, she had collected more than 2,000 prescriptions, including drugs for internal and external use, botanical drugs, and drugs made from animals and minerals. What's more, she screened more than 200 kinds of Chinese herbal medicines and more than 380 extracts mentioned in the prescriptions.

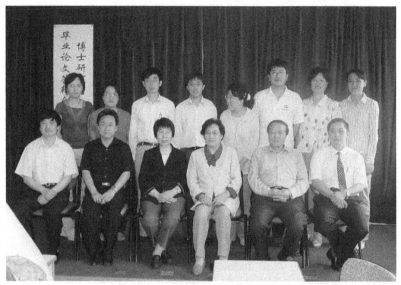

Tu Youyou (third from right in the front row) attends the graduate thesis defense of her PhD student Wang Manyuan (fourth from left in the back row). The teachers attending the thesis defense were: Huang Luqi (far right in the front row), head of the Institute of TCM; Sun Youfu (second from right in the front row), former director of the chemistry office at the Institute of TCM; Zhao Yuying (third from left in the front row), professor of the school of pharmacy at Peking University; Cui Chengbin (second from left in the front row), a researcher at the poisonous drug research institute at the Academy of Military Medical Sciences; Shi Renbing (far left in the front row), a professor of the school of TCM at Beijing University of Chinese Medicine

In 2002, Tu Youyou undertook subprojects about Artemisia apiacea that belonged to a special project named 'Standards of TCM and the related clinical efficacy evaluation of TCM'. However, the researcher Yang Lan, the sole group member, went to further his study in Japan. Due to the lack of researchers, Wang Manyuan, a new PhD student of Tu Youyou, was then instructed to join the research group. Each month, the 72-year-old Tu would take a taxi to the lab to guide him in his research work.

"Are you a doctor of Western medicine or TCM?" Wang Manyuan remembered asking Tu Youyou, but she never answered. As her student, he came to appreciate that Tu cared nothing about the arguments between TCM and Western medicine.

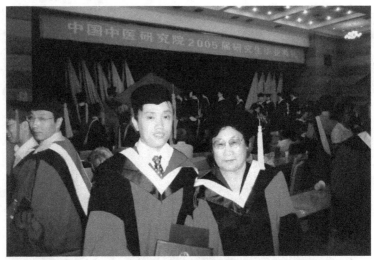

Tu Youyou and her PhD student Wang Manyuan at the 2005 graduation ceremony of postgraduates in the Chinese Academy of TCM

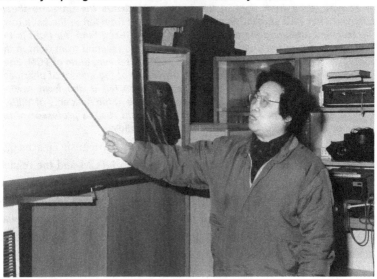

Tu Youyou reports on her project

"Her lifelong goal in scientific research is to improve the curative effect of TCM with the help of science and technology. That's also what she has taught me," said Wang Manyuan. At the beginning of his study, Wang received a 'gift' from Tu Youyou in the form of two master's papers written by her students Wu Chongming and Gu Yucheng. These two papers adopted Tu Youyou's research methods into artemisinin.

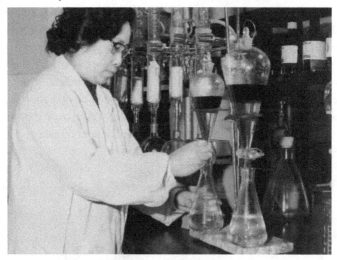

Tu Youyou conducts an experiment, February 1985

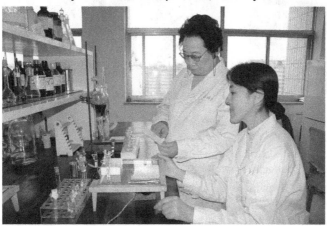

Tu Youyou guides her assistant Yang Lan in an experiment, 1996

In Wang's opinion, the gift allowed him to figure out not only the research idea but also the basis of Tu's research style.

When he was working hard on his doctoral degree, sponsored by Tu Youyou, Wang Manyuan also took courses in Chinese herbal medicine chemistry and wave spectrum analysis in Peking University Health Science Center and Peking University Medical College (PUMC).

"Professor Tu is quite persistent, decisive, career-oriented and single-minded," said Wang. What particularly impressed him was Tu Youyou's habit of keeping newspaper clippings on a daily basis. She paid special attention to events and news on health and often told him to search relevant information in order to enrich his knowledge. At the height of the SARS (sever acute respiratory syndrome) epidemic, and in co-operation with the Chinese Academy of Preventive Medicine, she researched the possible treatment effect of artemisinin-based drugs on the viral disease.

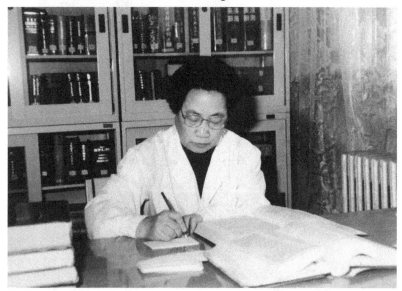

Tu Youyou conducts research

Wang Manyuan said: "Scientists of her generation had a strong commitment to the honor of the country, the sense of collective belonging, and the firm and pure scientific faith. She had an intangible but profound influence on me. It was from her that I learned that, once you settle on a research goal, you should firmly work for it on the road of scientific research."

Winning the Lasker Award

On September 12, 2011, Tu Youyou and her scientific research first came to public view.

On that day, the list of the 2011 Lasker award winners was announced and the Lasker-DeBakey clinical medical research award went to Tu Youyou for "the discovery of artemisinin, a drug therapy for malaria that has saved millions of lives across the globe, especially in developing countries".

Until the subsequent award of the Nobel prize, this was the highest global award ever won in the biomedical field in China.

Established to commend scientists, doctors and public service employees who have made prominent contributions in medicine, the Lasker award is second only to the Nobel prize in the biomedical field. Until 2011, when Tu Youyou won the award, dozens of the more than 300 Lasker award winners went on to win the Nobel prize. The importance of the Lasker awards is quite clear: announced before the Nobel prize, the Lasker award has gained a reputation for identifying future winners of the Nobel prize.

Thus, in the news reports on Tu Youyou at that time, the following comments were commonly heard: "Chinese woman closest ever to winning a Nobel prize" and "Worthy of winning the Nobel prize".

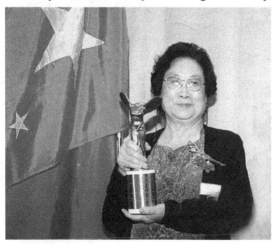

Tu wins the Lasker award, September 24, New York

Early in the morning of September 24, 2011, Tu Youyou received the trophy at the 2011 Lasker awards ceremony. At the age of 81, she gave an earnest speech: "This is an honor that brings Chinese medicine to the world. It belongs to everyone in the research team, and it belongs to all TCM scientists. "

Indeed, it was the first time that people from across the world knew that the time-honored TCM and TCM pharmacology had successfully conquered a worldwide health problem.

"Not often in the history of clinical medicine can we celebrate a discovery that has eased the pain and distress of hundreds of millions of people and saved countless lives in more than 100 countries," said the Lasker awards jury member and professor of Stanford University, Lucy Shapiro, while describing the significance of Tu's discovery. The discovery of artemisinin, a highly effective anti-malarial drug, was largely due to the "scientific insight, vision and dogged determination" of Tu and her team, and has provided the world with arguably the most important pharmaceutical intervention therapy in the past half-century.

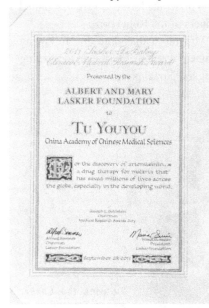
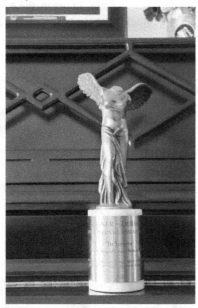

The Lasker award certificate and trophy

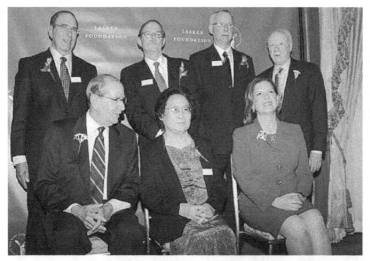

Tu Youyou along with judges and winners of the 2011 Lasker award. In addition to Tu, the other individual winners were Arthur L. Horwich (second from left in the back row) and Franz-Ulrich Hartl (third from left in the back row). The Clinical Center of the National Institutes of Health received the Lasker-Bloomberg public service award as an organization; its honoree stands far left in the back row

The coordinator of the WHO global malaria program, Pascal Ringwald, said that, over the previous 10 years, the global death toll due to malaria had fallen by 38%. And in 43 countries, including 11 in Africa, the incidence and death rate of malaria had fallen by more than 50%. The advent of artemisinin-based drugs improved the weaponry in their battle against malaria.

Aside from the anti-malarial efficacy of artemisinin, Tu Youyou was particularly concerned about the significance of winning this award for TCM and TCM pharmacology. At the awards ceremony, after calmly describing the development process of artemisinin, Tu Youyou said with excitement: "We call for the further exploration of TCM, and also TCM innovation, improvement and legacy. TCM and TCM pharmacology is a great treasure and its potential for people's health worldwide merits further exploration. Considerable experience has been left by our ancestors and the discovery of artemisinin has helped solve a global problem. Yet, there are still many other useful medicines worth being explored. "

In the letter of congratulation to Tu, the State Administration of TCM said that her winning of the Lasker award demonstrated that TCM and TCM pharmacology were a great treasure and of great value, and that Chinese science and innovation of science and technology in the biomedical field were of great value, which inspired many TCM professionals.

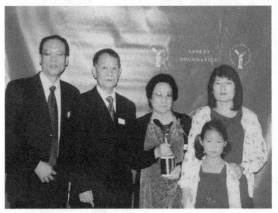

Tu Youyou, her husband and the family members of her elder daughter Li Min at the Lasker award ceremony, September 2011

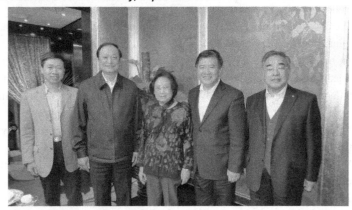

November 2011: Chen Zhu, Minister of Health (second from right); Wang Guoqiang Vice-Minister of Health and director of the State Administration of Traditional Chinese Medicine (second from left); Wang Zhiyong secretary of the party committee of the CACMS (left); Zhang Boli, dean of the China Academy of Chinese Medical Sciences (right), and Tu Youyou, three months after winning the Lasker award

After learning that Tu Youyou had won the Lasker award, Rao Yi, dean of the PKU school of life science, who studied the history of artemisinin, said: "Domestic and international efforts in researching TCM may bring it into a new era and save more lives." The discovery of artemisinin has proven the value of obtaining certain chemical drugs from traditional medicine and it can stimulate international medical circles to find drugs with new chemical structures and effective compounds from traditional medicines. It also encourages scientists to endeavor to identify the relationship between specific chemical components of TCM and specific diseases.

Artemisinin is still benefiting humans. This scientific achievement rooted in the land of China, a treasure of TCM and TCM pharmacy, has received more and more authoritative affirmation in international biomedical circles since Tu Youyou won the Lasker award.

Four years after winning the award, Tu and her team were again recognized by scientists on the international stage. In June 2015, she and two other scientists were given the Warren Alpert prize for their pioneering and innovative contributions to the prevention and cure of malaria. Tu was unable to attend the ceremony because of her physical condition, so her family members represented her instead.

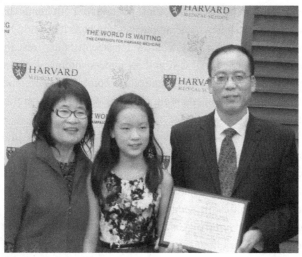

Tu Youyou's elder daughter Li Min, son-in-law Mao Lei and granddaughter accepted the Warren Alpert prize on her behalf

The Warren Alpert Foundation was established in 1987 by Mr Warren Alpert with the aim of honoring scientists who make breakthroughs in human health. So far, it has been awarded to 51 scientists, of whom eight (including Tu Youyou) have gone on to receive the Nobel prize. Tu Youyou was the first Chinese scientist to receive the Warren Alpert award.

Unexpected Nobel Prize

On October 5, 2015, four years after winning the Lasker award, sometimes known as the 'weather vane of the Nobel prize', Tu Youyou became a real Nobel prize winner.

On that day, the Karolinska Institute in Sweden announced that the 2015 Nobel prize in physiology or medicine had been awarded to the Chinese medical scientist Tu Youyou, the Irish scientist William Campbell and the Japanese scientist Satoshi Ōmura to commend their achievements in therapeutic research into parasitic diseases.

Thus, in "discovering a new therapy against malaria", Tu Youyou became the 12th female winner in the history of the Nobel prize in physiology or medicine. Jean Anderson, judge of the Nobel prize in physiology or medicine, said: "Tu Youyou was the first scientist to confirm that artemisinin can be effective against malaria for both human beings and animals. Her research has made an outstanding contribution to human life and health, and opened a new window for scientists and researchers. Tu Youyou has knowledge of TCM and an understanding of pharmacology and chemistry as well. She has managed to combine eastern and western medicine, and achieved outstanding results. Her findings were the perfect combination of both."

The Nobel prize committee described the achievements of the 2015 winners as "immeasurable": "Diseases caused by parasites have plagued humankind for thousands of years, resulting in a severe global health concern. The application of artemisinin discovered by Tu Youyou in her treatments has significantly reduced the mortality rate of malaria patients, and abamectin discovered by Campbell and Ōmura has ultimately reduced the incidence of river blindness and lymphatic filariasis. This year's prize-winners have formulated 'revolutionary treatments to the most damaging parasitic diseases'. These two achievements provide 'new effective treatments' for millions of people infected by these diseases every year, and they are immeasurable accomplishments for improving human health and reducing the pain of patients."

During the National Day holidays in 2015, all Chinese people were delighted for Tu Youyou's success.

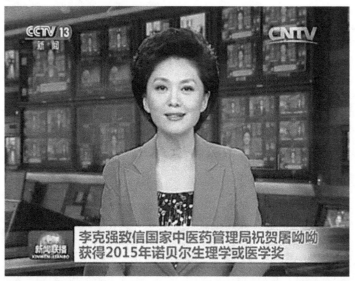

Premier Li Keqiang sent a letter of congratulations to Tu Youyou for winning the 2015 Nobel prize in physiology or medicine. The story was covered on CCTV News on October 6

On the day when the news was announced, Li Keqiang, member of the standing committee of the political bureau of the CPC central committee and premier of the State Council, sent a letter to the State Administration of TCM to congratulate the famous Chinese pharmaceutical scientist Tu Youyou on winning the 2015 Nobel prize in physiology or medicine. Li wrote in his letter that, for a long time, many scientific and technical workers in our country, including medical researchers, have been working silently, contributing selflessly, collaborating and scaling new heights, and have attained a host of high-level achievements. Tu's success represents China's prosperity and progress in the fields of science and technology, reflects TCM's huge contribution to human health and fully demonstrates the constant improvement of China's comprehensive national power and international influence. He expressed the hope that many more scientific researchers would conscientiously implement the strategy of innovation-driven development, actively promote mass entrepreneurship and innovation, explore the frontiers of science and technology, and endeavor to conquer difficulties to make new and greater contributions to promoting domestic social and economic development, and speeding up the construction of an innovative country.

On the evening of October 5, 2015, Liu Yandong, member of the political bureau of the CPC central committee and vice-premier of the State Council, asked the China Association of Science and Technology and the State Administration of TCM to visit Tu Youyou and express his congratulations.

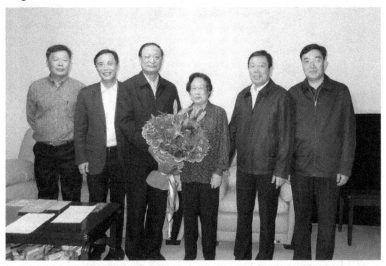

On the evening on October 5, 2015, entrusted by Vice-Premier Liu Yandong, Shang Yong (second from right), party secretary of the China Association for Science and Technology, Wang Guoqiang (third from left), director of the State Administration of TCM, and others, visited Tu Youyou

On October 5, the All-China Women's Federation sent a letter to Tu Youyou congratulating her on winning the 2015 Nobel prize in physiology or medicine; on the afternoon of October 10, the vice-chair of the standing committee of the National People's Congress (NPC) and president of the All-China Women's Federation, Shen Yueyue, visited Tu Youyou.

Several national authorities held related forums. On October 8, at a joint forum held by the National Health and Family Planning Commission of the PRC, the State Administration of TCM and the China Food and Drug Administration congratulating Tu Youyou on winning the 2015 Nobel prize, Chen Zhu, vice-chairman of the standing committee of the NPC, expressed his congratulations to Tu. He said Tu's work laid the most important foundation for the treatment of human malaria by artemisinin and was vigorously promoted by our country and the WHO. Her work also helped save millions of lives of people suffering from malaria around the world, especially in developing countries, making a great contribution to controlling and finding a cure for this major parasitic infectious disease. Moreover, it had become the most brilliant example of promoting the inheritance and innovation of TCM in a scientific way and demonstrating the importance of TCM to the world. As a fellow scientist with international influence, Chen Zhu also cared for and supported artemisinin research, and pointed out that artemisinin was the pride of China.

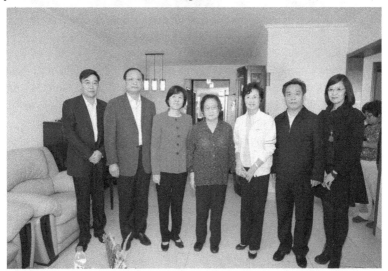

On the afternoon of October 10, Shen Yueyue (third from left), vice-chair of the standing committee of the NPC and president of the All-China Women's Federation, Song Xiuyan (third from right), party secretary of the All-China Women's Federation, and Wang Guoqiang (second from left), director of the State Administration of TCM, and others visited Tu Youyou

On October 8, the China Association of Science and Technology also held a forum entitled 'The scientific community congratulates Tu Youyou on winning the Nobel prize in medicine'...

Tu Youyou's achievement also aroused widespread international interest.

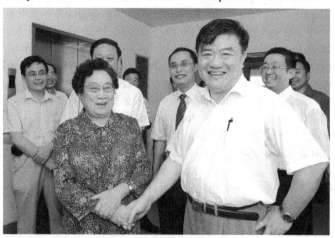

Chen Zhu visits Tu Youyou

Why did Tu Youyou win this award?

In the 60 years since she was assigned to work at the Institute of Chinese Materia Medica of the CACMS in 1955, Tu Youyou has seldom left her office. She has spent her time focusing on those amazing 'Chinese herbs' in which she achieved such excellent results.

After finding artemisinin, Tu Youyou didn't stop there. Her persistent work ethic drove her to explore further. In 1973, she synthesized dihydroartemisinin to prove the existence of carbonyl in artemisinin; the chemical substance she synthesized later was proven to have a much stronger effect than natural artemisinin.

With the combined efforts of Tu Youyou and her research group, they finished their research into artemisinin suppositories by August 1983. In 1986, a new drug certificate was given for artemisinin with the code (86) WYSZx-01.

This was the first new drug certificate issued by the Ministry of Health since the *Pharmaceutical Administration Law of the PRC* and *Rules for New Drug Examination and Approval* in 1985.

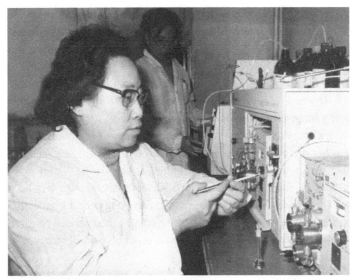

In the 1990s, Tu Youyou conducted the liquid phase analysis test of dihydroartemisinin

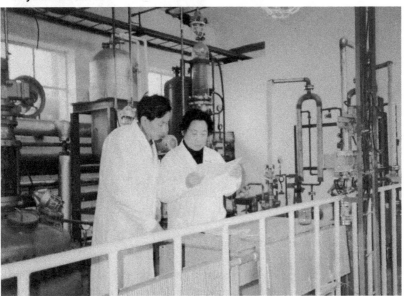

Tu Youyou guides a technician in Beijing No. 6 Pharmaceutical Factory, 1992

From September 1973, when three cases of artemisinin capsules were found to be fully effective in clinical preliminary tests, to 1986 when artemisinin products were first officially launched onto the market, nearly 13 years had passed!

Immersed in research into Chinese herbal medicines, Tu Youyou wrote and edited *Artemisia Annua and Artemisinin-based Drug*s in 2009. It was subsequently included in the 11th five-year plan list of 'national important books'. She always tells visitors that this book, an academic work of 260 pages, was her preferred way to present herself to the world as a scientist; as for other things, she seemed to have nothing to say.

It can be seen from Tu Youyou's published works that she has been focusing on the Chinese herb Artemisia annua for a long period, conducting research into its effective components. She has published various research achievements on authentic Artemisia annua products and derivatives of Artemisia annua.

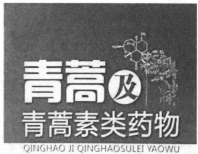

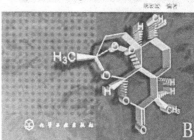

The front cover of Tu Youyou's Artemisia Annua and Artemisinin-based Drugs

Though Tu Youyou didn't possess a grand title, this did not prevent her from dedicating herself to the medical field and eventually winning the Nobel prize.

She said: "I've researched artemisinin for my whole life, so I hope we can make the best use of it, and I wish for a new incentive mechanism to help TCM make more valuable achievements and play a greater role in protecting human health."

The originality and innovative superiority of TCM was also an important assistance for To Youyou to win the Nobel prize.

In fact, TCM has always been China's scientific and technical area with great original innovative superiority.

Zhang Zhongjing of the Eastern Han dynasty was famous for treating 'typhia', and his traditional Chinese medical classic *Shanghan Lun* (*Treatise on Febrile Diseases*) discusses therapies for numerous infectious diseases in different periods. The prescriptions contained in this book are still in use today. Its flexible and dialectic therapies laid the foundation for the clinical practice of TCM. The classical school of Chinese medicine in Japan still uses Zhang's original prescriptions for the treatment of viral hepatitis and other infections.

From 980 to 1567, before the invention of the cowpox vaccination, the Chinese invention of variolation was the most effective way to prevent smallpox. It was used extensively in China, then later entered Europe and became popular in the US, saving millions of lives and promoting the birth of modern immune preventive medicine.

From 369 BC to 1644 AD in the late Ming dynasty, 95 pandemics were recorded in China's official history. In documents that record the history of the Qing dynasty, there were more than 100 pandemics. Despite such a high incidence of pandemics, the population in China in those years grew rapidly. In the middle of the Qing dynasty, the population was more than 100m, and in the late Qing dynasty it reached 300m, while Europe's population at the time was just 150m and growing slowly. There are many possible reasons for this, but the contribution of TCM is undeniable.

From Tu Youyou's point of view, the significance of discovering artemisinin was in connecting with the past: "I am particularly glad that I discovered the essence of our ancestors through modern pharmacy."

Behind that idea lies the most popular saying in TCM circles in China: "Combining traditional Chinese medicine and western medicine".

As a student in the third session of the national class for learning TCM after studying western medicine, Tu Youyou's scientific research methods are without parallel.

This female scientist growing up in the early years of the new China was very clear about this time when the whole country was promoting "combining traditional Chinese medicine and western medicine", which had great significance for the development of TCM.

Nowadays, TCM receives more recognition from the international community. As the chairman of the Nobel Committee for Physiology or Medicine said: "Chinese female scientist Tu Youyou's application of artemisinin extracted from TCM for the treatment of malaria indicates that traditional Chinese herbal medicines can also bring scientists new inspiration." She added that, through their combination of modern extraction technology and modern medicine, Chinese herbal medicines have made "great" achievements in the treatment of diseases.

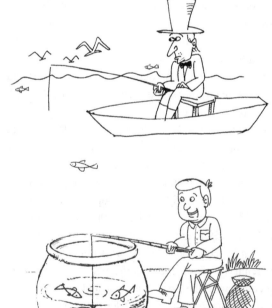

In the research and development of new drugs in the west, listed drug compounds are screened from hundreds of thousands of compounds, a process that is just like fishing in the sea. Traditional Chinese medicine has a history of thousands of years and its modern R&D is to fish in the pond of TCM

Chinese culture is profound and extensive. TCM is the creation and accumulation of Chinese civilization over thousands of years and a great treasure house that needs to be inherited. The existence of TCM has protected the health of countless Chinese people. It has been a superb global medicine for a very long time. The legendary ancient doctors Bian Que and Hua Tuo both reflected on the splendor of TCM in certain historical periods. Today, Tu Youyou's Nobel prize reaffirms its potential. It is imperative that we retain the legacy of TCM.

Zhang Boli, president of the CACMS and academician of the Chinese Academy of Engineering, was struck by this point of view. He thought that the combination of TCM's original thinking with modern science and technology could result in original achievements. After learning that Tu had been awarded the Nobel prize in physiology or medicine, he said: "TCM is never isolated from external influence. It changes with the times, developing continuously and absorbing the new knowledge and technical methods of different times. At present, with the rapid progress of science and technology, TCM should develop in combination with modern technology so as to enrich its scientific content and characteristics. TCM is a primary area with proprietary intellectual property rights in China. Its unique theoretical system and original thinking is an endless source of scientific and technological innovation, containing great innovative potential. The successful research and development of artemisinin abides by this principle that the combination of TCM's original thinking with modern science and technology can result in original achievements. The advocation to modernize TCM does not mean that tradition is less important. The approaches of scientific and technological innovation of TCM not only lie in seeking inspiration from ancient medical books, but also in learning from advanced science and technology. The combination of TCM and modern technology theories and methods enriches the life sciences, enhances medical and health services, contributes to the implementation of innovative strategies and changes the economic development pattern."

As for the superior originality of TCM, the director of the Institute of Chinese Materia Medica of the CACMS, Chen Shilin, said: "Anything with a stronger national spirit is more vigorous. Great original science and technology resources lie in the field of traditional medicine combine' with modern science and technology, possibly producing many original and significant research achievements and thereby benefiting humans. For example, arsenic (As2O3) used in the treatment of leukemia, tetrandrine used in antiviral therapy, berberine used in the treatment of diabetes and so on."

In addition, we should pay special attention to the fact that it was a woman who won the first Nobel prize in the natural sciences field in China. This was an amazing and exciting achievement!

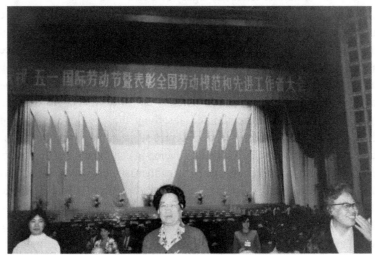

Tu Youyou attends the '5.1' International Workers' Day and Chinese National Model Workers and Advanced Workers Awards Ceremony, 1995

In the 115 years since the establishment of the Nobel prize, there have been 592 prize-winning scientists in natural sciences, 17 of whom were women, accounting for just 3% of the total. Among them, there have been only four female winners of the Nobel prize in chemistry, including Marie Curie and her daughter, Irène Joliot Curie. There were only two female winners of the Nobel prize in physics, one of whom was, again, Marie Curie. Th____ ' ve been no female winners of the Nobel prize in physics
           situation is better for the Nobel prize in physiology or
           there have been 12 female winners, but they only account
           tal. Against such a historical background, Tu Youyou's
           el prize in physiology or medicine is not only a source of

pride in scientific circles in China but also the pride of Chinese women and women the world over.

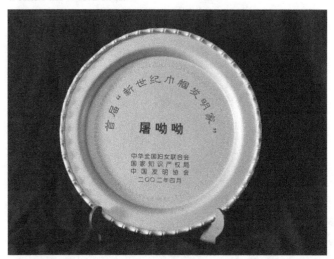

In April 2002, Tu Youyou was named among the 'Women Inventors in the New Century' awarded by the All-China Women's Federation, the State Intellectual Property Office and the China Association of Inventors

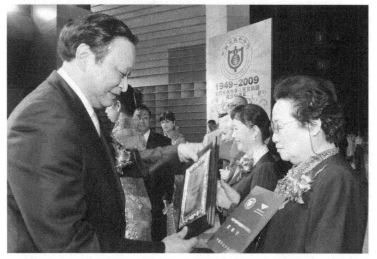

Tu Youyou receives the Tang TCM development award of the CACMS, 2009. The award was founded by Cyrus Chung Ying Tang

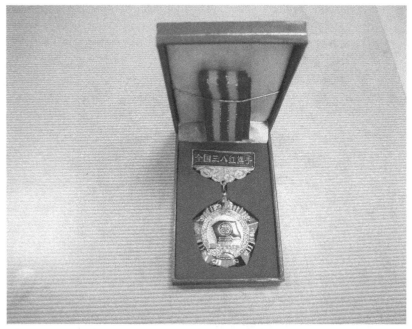

In February 2012, Tu Youyou won the National 'March 8th' Red Banner awarded by the All-China Women's Federation

Tu Youyou's triumph indicates that Chinese women are outstandingly intelligent. Her career shows that, after successfully 'walking out of the kitchen', women have stepped onto a huge stage. With great ability and potential in scientific research, women have proved that the old-fashioned stereotype of women being inferior in the scientific research field is no more than prejudiced nonsense.

Tu Youyou's experiences fully show that the series of gender equality policies implemented in the new China have played a role in both promoting female empowerment and national development. Her Nobel prize is the greatest achievement of the women's emancipation movement in the new China. With the country paying increasing attention to nurturing female talent, the introduction of more policies and measures supporting their growth and all sectors of society jointly creating an environment beneficial for their development, more and more 'Tu Youyous' will emerge in an equitable environment and prosper in a space without 'glass ceilings'.

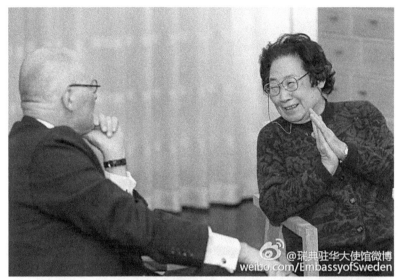

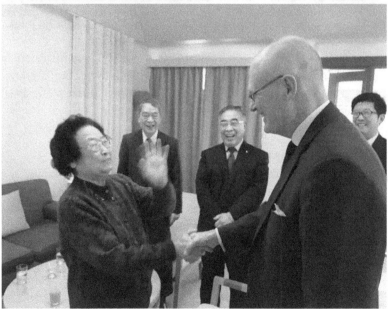

Tu Youyou talks with Lars Freden, Sweden's ambassador to China, about receiving the Nobel prize in Sweden, November 19, 2015

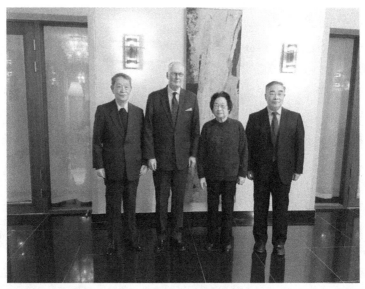

Tu Youyuo with her husband Li Tingzhao, Zhang Boli, director of the CACMS and academician of the Chinese Academy of Engineering, and Lars Peter Fredén, Sweden's ambassador to China, November 19, 2015

Now, at the age of 85, Tu Youyou is still obsessed with her career in TCM. This respectable woman fully reflects the lofty medical workers' spirit of serving the public and saving lives, fully embodies the professional demeanor of being pragmatic, determined to explore, devoted to one's career and courageous in innovation.

Stubborn Youyou

In 2005, Tu Youyou's family moved from Sanlitun to a tall building in a residential area of Beijing, near Jintai Road, Chaoyang district. It is a typical Beijing apartment with a living room, dining room and three bedrooms. The apartment's wide view not only brings fine sunlight, but also offers a full view of the headquarters of CCTV, the People's Daily building and other new landmarks in Beijing, all from the living room. Tu Youyou and her husband were quite satisfied with their new apartment. In accordance with her family's custom, it was naturally her husband, Li Tingzhao, who had the final say over this important purchasing decision. In his later years, Li regarded the apartment as one of his most satisfying work spaces. It was right here that Tu Youyou won the international awards that made her a world-renowned figure.

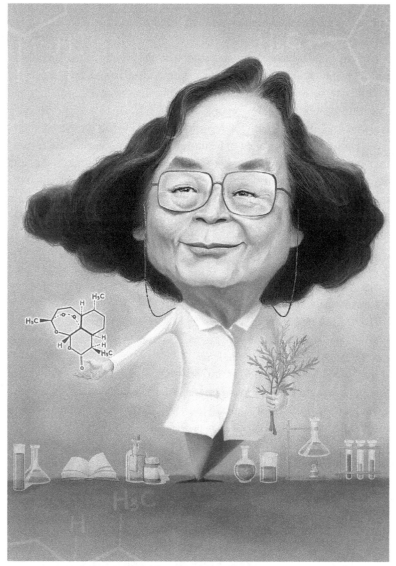

A cartoon of Tu Youyou (drawn and provided by Cao Yi)

Even in her 80s, Tu Youyou never regarded herself as retired. This is not merely because she is a life-long researcher at China Academy of TCM and director of the Artemisinin Research Center. More important, her personal interest in medicine has never wavered since her college days due to her stubborn character.

As artemisinin has become more popular and widely used, Tu Youyou shifted her attention to artemisinin abuse and the plasmodium's resistance to artemisinin. She noticed that the problems were mentioned in some scientific papers and news reports. Artemisinin used as a special anti-malarial drug was gradually taking a longer cycle to kill the plasmodium. Even worse, some types of artemisinin-resistant plasmodiums had appeared in malaria-stricken areas. Like other researchers in this field, Tu was deeply worried about the appearance of artemisinin-resistant plasmodiums mentioned in the recent reports. To solve the problem, the WHO made a strategic decision to stop recommending the sole use of artemisinin for malaria treatment.

She also mentioned that the massive use of artemisinin in certain areas is one of the potential causes of medicine resistance. She hoped that malaria treatment would be standardized worldwide and that the abuse of artemisinin would be prohibited.

Tu Youyou was frank in her view on how to use artemisinin. No matter what others said and did, she always tried to stick to her point of view. She never changed her stubborn character.

In 1975, she was criticized for her stubbornness at a conference in Chengdu that aimed to further research on artemisinin. According to the records of 'Mission 523' (from 1964 to 1981) by Li Runhong, the research institutions reported their research process at this conference. Particular mention was made of the research team from Guangdong province's TCM Institute, who had made significant achievements during their eight-year-long investigation in malarial areas and gained rich experiences in treating cerebral malaria. Some other research institutions tended to conduct their research only in the laboratory, with their door closed. According to informed sources, Tu Youyou's research team was among the targets of those critical words. At that time, when more and more people were passionately focusing on clinical trials on artemisinin, Tu Youyou, as the discoverer of artemisinin, insisted that its chemical construction should first be identified in the lab, and then put it into a large-scale clinical application. She thought that this was the correct approach to adopt for the sake of patients and to follow the basic law of medicine.

Closely related with her stubbornness is her dogged pursuit and appreciation for innovation. On the evening of December 2, just two days before her departure for Stockholm to receive the Nobel prize, Tu Youyou talked about the importance of innovation with Chen Shilin, director of the Institute of Chinese Materia Medicine affiliated to the Chinese Academy of TCM. Li Tingzhao, Tu Youyou's husband, interjected: "Innovation has already been included in the fifth plenary session and written in the relevant documents."

On hearing this, she said in a strong voice: "What a wise decision the central committee has made! I approve." She then continued: "In fact, discovering the secret of artemisinin was also an act of innovation at that time. We had tried various means. Now it still needs continuous innovation to rejuvenate artemisinin's vitality." For Tu Youyou, who is already 85 years old, innovation is no longer a fashionable word but a concept that she has been practicing all along and a key factor on the road to her success in scientific research.

Her stubborn character is also reflected in her deep patriotic feelings. Whenever the country is in need, Tu Youyou will try her best to accomplish the task. The earnest love for her country is what she cherishes most. In order to undertake the mission of artemisinin research, she chose, without hesitation, to separate from her two daughters. In order to understand the toxic effects of the artemisinin, she risked her own life to test the medicine on herself.

After reviewing the significant decisions and choices that a woman over 80 has made, we can always find the determining factor: serving the country. The same is true of her decision to go to Sweden to receive the Noble prize. Tu Youyou was originally hesitant about whether to make the journey because of her advanced age, poor health and particularly a strain in her lower back. She had expressed this attitude clearly when she was interviewed by the *New York Times* and other media. However, her colleagues said that the Nobel prize was not only her personal honor but also a national glory, and that she had better go if she could; on that basis, she immediately decided to go to Sweden. Li said whenever the country needs her, she is always there. This is typical of her.

Being stubborn about the rules, innovation, patriotism and pursuing her dream, Tu Youyou marches forward courageously in spite of numerous difficulties and dangers. That's Tu Youyou, a Chinese scientist with a unique and deep emotion.

Appendix

Speech by Tu Youyou at the Karolinska Institutet in Sweden

(December 7, 2015)

Dear respected chairman, general secretary, esteemed Nobel laureates, ladies and gentlemen.

It is my great honor to give this lecture today at the Karolinska Institutet. The title of my presentation is 'Artemisinin – A Gift from Traditional Chinese Medicine to the World'.

Before starting, I would like to thank the Nobel Assembly and the Nobel Foundation for awarding me the 2015 Nobel prize in physiology or medicine. It is not only an honor for me, but also recognition and motivation for all scientists in China. I would also like to express my sincere appreciation for the great hospitality that I have received from the Swedish people during my short stay over the last few days.

Thanks to Dr William Campbell and Dr Satoshi Ōmura for their excellent and inspiring presentations. The story I will tell today is of the diligent and dedicated Chinese scientists searching for anti-malarial drugs from traditional Chinese medicines 40 years ago under arduous and inadequate research conditions.

Some of you may have read the history of artemisinin's discovery in numerous publications. I will give a brief review. The diagram here summarizes the anti-malarial research program carried out by the team at the Institute of Chinese Materia Medica (ICMM) of the Academy of Traditional Chinese Medicine (ATCM).

The programs highlighted in blue were accomplished by the team at the the ATCM, while the un-highlighted programs were completed collaboratively by other research teams across the nation. The programs highlighted in blue and white were completed through joint efforts by the teams at the ATCM and other institutes.

Summary of the Work Completed by the Research Team in Academy of Traditional Chinese Medicine (Boxes in Blue Background)

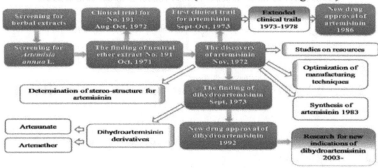

The team at the ICMM initiated research on TCMs for malaria treatment in 1969. Following substantial screening, we started in 1971 to focus on the herb *qinghao* (sweet wormwood), which is Chinese for Artemisia annua, but received no promising results despite multiple attempts. In September 1971, a modified procedure was designed to reduce the extraction temperature by immersing or distilling *qinghao* using ethyl ether, and the obtained extracts were then treated with an alkaline solution to remove acidic impurities and retain the neutral portion. In the experiments carried out on October 4 1971, sample No. 191, the neutral portion of the *qinghao* ether extract was found 100% effective on malaria-infected mice by peroral treatment at a dose of 1g/kg for three consecutive days. The same results were observed when tested on malaria-infected monkeys from December 1971 to January 1972. So the breakthrough finding of the neutral portion of the *qinghao* ether extract became a crucial step in discovering artemisinin.

We subsequently carried out a clinical trial from August to October 1972 in which the neutral *qinghao* ether extract successfully cured 30 falciparum and plasmodium malaria-affected patients. In November 1972, an effective antimalarial compound was isolated from the neutral *qinghao* ether extract. The compound was later named *qinghaosu* (artemisinin).

We started to determine the chemical structure of artemisinin in

December 1972 through elemental analysis, spectrophotometry, mass spectrum, polarimetric analysis and other techniques. These experiments confirmed that the compound had a complete new sesquiterpene structure with a formula of $C_{15}H_{22}O_5$, a molecular weight of 282 and containing no nitrogen.

The formula of the molecule and other results were verified by the analytical chemistry department of the China Academy of Medical Sciences on April 27, 1973.

We started collaboration with the Shanghai Institute of Organic Chemistry and the Institute of Biophysics of the CAS on artemisinin chemical structure analysis in 1974. The stereo-structure was finally determined using the X-ray diffraction technique which verified that artemisinin was a new sesquiterpenelactone containing a peroxy group. The structure was published in 1977 and cited by the publication *Chemical Abstracts.*

Molecular Structure of Artemisinin and its Derivatives

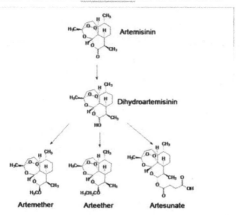

Derivatization of artemisinin was performed in 1973 in order to determine its functional group. A carboxyl group was verified in the artemisnin molecule through reduction by sodium borohydride. Dihydroartemisinin was found in this process. Further research on the structure-activity relationship of artemisinin was conducted. The peroxyl group in the artemisnin molecule was proven crucial for its antimalarial function. Efficacy was improved for some compounds derivatized through the hydroxy group of dihydroartemisinin.

Here we show the chemical structures of artemisinin and its derivatives, which are dihydroartemisinin, artemether, artesunate and arteether. Up to now, no clinical application has been reported with other artemisinin derivatives except for the four presented here.

The Artemisinin new drug certificate and Dihydroartemisinin new drug certificate were granted by China's Ministry of Health in 1986 and 1992, respectively. Dihydroartemisinin is 10 times more potent than artemisinin, again demonstrated 'high efficacy, rapid action and low toxicity' of the drugs in the artemisnin category.

In 1981, the WHO, World Bank and United Nations Development Program held the fourth joint malaria chemotherapy science working group meeting in Beijing. A series of presentations on artemisinin and its clinical application including my report *Studies on the Chemistry of Qinghaosu* received positive and enthusiastic responses. In the 1980s, thousands of malaria-affected patients were cured with artemisinin and its derivatives in China.

After this brief review, you may believe that this is no more than an ordinary drug discovery process. However, it was neither simple nor easy to discover artemisinin from *qinghao*, a Chinese herb medicine with a clinical application of more than 2,000 years.

The ICMM of the ATCM joined the national 'Mission 523' anti-malaria research project in 1969. I was appointed head by the academy's leadership to build the 'Mission 523' research group in the institute and to be responsible for developing new antimalarial drugs from Chinese medicines. It was a confidential military program with high priority. As a young scientist early in my career, I felt overwhelmed by the trust and responsibility inherent in such a challenging and important task. I made up my mind to fully devote myself to accomplishing my duties.

The photo below was taken soon after I joined the ICMM. On the left, Professor Lou Zhicen, a famous pharmacognosist, was mentoring me on how to differentiate herbs. From 1959 to 1962, I attended a training course on theories and practices of TCM designed for professionals with a modern (western) medicine training background. The French chemist Louis Pasteur once said: "Fortune favors the prepared mind." There is also an old saying: "What's past is prologue." However, my prologue is a kind of integrated

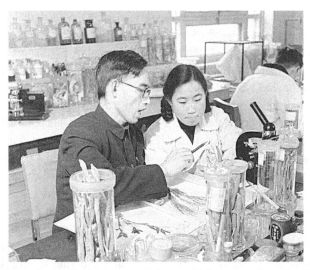

training in modern and Chinese medicines, which prepared me for rising to the challenge when the opportunities in searching for anti-malarial Chinese medicine became available.

After accepting the tasks, I collected more than 2,000 herbal, animal and mineral prescriptions for either internal or external use through reviewing ancient traditional Chinese medical literature and folk recipes, interviewing well-known and experienced Chinese medical doctors who provided me with prescriptions and herbal recipes. I summarized 640 prescriptions in the brochure *Antimalarial Collections of Recipes and Prescriptions*. It was the information collection and deciphering that laid sound foundation for the discovery of artemisinin. It also differentiates the approaches taken by Chinese medicine and general phytochemistry in searching for novel drugs.

I reviewed the literature about TCM when our research stalled following numerous failures. In reading Ge Hong's *A Handbook of Prescriptions for Emergencies* (from the Eastern Jin dynasty, in the 4th-5th century), I further digested the sentence "A handful of *qinghao* immersed in two liters of water, wring out the juice and drink it all" when *qinghao* was mentioned for alleviating malaria symptoms. It reminded me that the heating process might need to be avoided during extraction; thus, the method was modified by using a solvent with a low boiling point.

The earliest mention of *qinghao's* application as a herbal medicine was found in the silk manuscript *Prescriptions for 52 Kinds of Disease* unearthed from the third Han tomb at Mawangdui in Changsha, Hunan province. Its medical application was also recorded in *Shen Nong's Herbal Classic, Bu Yi Lei Gong Bao Zhi* and *Compendium of Materia Medica*. However, no clear botanical classification was given for *qinghao* despite the many references to the name in this literature. At this time, all species in the *qinghao* family were mixed. Two species were collected in *Chinese Pharmacopoeia* and four others were also being prescribed. Our subsequent investigation proved that only Artemisia annua L contained artemisinin and was effective against malaria, which exacerbated the task of discovering artemisinin. Apart from the confusion in finding the right plant, variables such as the part and origin of the plant, its harvest season, low artemisinin content in the plant, and the extraction and purification process, added extra difficulty in the discovery. Success in identifying the effectiveness of *qinghao* neutral ether extract is not easy. Thus, TCM contains rich resources, which need to be explored and improved upon.

In the 1970s, research conditions were relatively poor in China, so our team had to use household water vats for extraction to produce a sufficient quantity of *qinghao* extract for clinical trial. Some team members' health deteriorated due to exposure to a large quantity of organic solvent and insufficient ventilation equipment. In order to launch a clinical trial sooner while not compromising patient safety, based on the limited safety data from the animal study, the team members and I volunteered to take *qinghao* extract ourselves to determine its safety. When unsatisfactory results were observed in the clinical trial using artemisinin tablets, the team carried out a thorough investigation and verified poor disintegration of the tablets as the root cause. This allowed us to quickly resume the trial using capsules and find artemisinin's clinical efficacy in time.

An anti-malarial drug research symposium was held by the national 'Mission 523' office in Nanjing on March 8, 1972. In the meeting, on behalf of the ICMM, I reported the positive readouts of *qinghao* extract No. 191 observed in animal studies performed on malaria-affected mice and monkeys. The presentation received significant attention. On November 17, 1972, I reported the success of the 30 clinical cases at the national conference held in Beijing, which led to a nationwide collaboration in researching *qinghao* for anti-malaria treatment.

Today, I would like to express my sincere appreciation again to my fellow colleagues in the ATCM for their devotion and exceptional contributions to 'Mission 523' during the discovery and subsequent application of artemisinin. Once again, I would like to thank and congratulate the colleagues from Shandong Provincial Institute of Chinese Medicine, Yunnan Provincial Institute of Materia Medica, the Institute of Biophysics of Chinese Academy of Sciences, Shanghai Institute of Organic Chemistry of the Chinese Academy of Sciences, Guangzhou University of Chinese Medicine, the Academy of Military Medical Sciences and many other institutes for their invaluable contributions in different areas during collaboration and their care for malaria patients. I would also like to express my sincere respect to the 'Mission 523' office leadership for their continuous efforts in organizing and coordinating the anti-malarial research programs. Without collective effort, we would not be able to present artemisinin to the world in such a short period of time.

"The findings in this year's *World Malaria Report* demonstrate that the world is continuing to make impressive progress in reducing malaria cases and deaths," said Dr Margaret Chan, director-general of the WHO when referring to controlling malaria. But statistically, there are about 3.3bn people across 97 countries or regions still at risk of malaria infection and around 1.2bn living in high-risk areas where the infection rate is as high as more than 1 per 1,000. Statistics show that, in 2013, there were about 198m people affected with malaria globally and about 580,000 people died from it. Around 78% of those who died were children under five. Nine in 10 malaria deaths occur in Africa, and 70% of African malaria-affected patients receive artemisinin combination therapies (ACTs); however, as many as 56m-69m children affected with malaria do not have ACTs available to them.

P. falciparum resistance to artemisinin has been detected in five countries of the Greater Mekong sub-region, including Cambodia, Laos, Myanmar, Thailand and Vietnam. In many areas along the Cambodia-Thailand border, P. falciparum has become resistant to most available anti-malaria medicines, which is a severe warning since resistance to artemisinin has also appeared in some African regions.

The WHO put forward a global plan for artemisinin resistant containment (GPARC) in 2011, and its goal is to protect ACTs as an effective treatment for P. falciparum malaria. Artemisinin resistance has been confirmed within the Greater Mekong sub-region, and potential epidemic risk is under critical review. More than 100 experts involved in the program thought that the chance of containing and eradicating artemisinin-resistant malaria was very limited before the resistance to the medicine spread to highly-affected areas, and it was urgent to constrain artemisinin resistance. To protect the efficacy of ACT, I strongly suggest a global compliance to the GPARC performed by all the scientists and medical doctors in the field.

Before I conclude my lecture, I would like to briefly discuss something about TCM: "Chinese medicine and pharmacology are a great treasure. We should explore and raise them to a higher level." These words are engraved on the front gate of the China Academy of Chinese Medical Sciences. Artemisinin was explored from the treasure that is Chinese medicine. From our experience in researching artemisinin, we felt deeply that both Chinese and western medicines had their strengths. There are great potential and development prospects if these strengths can be fully integrated. We have substantial plant resources from nature so that our fellow medical researchers can develop brand-new medicines from them. Considerable clinical experience has been accumulated in the development of TCM over thousands of years since the time when Shennong [the Chinese Emperor of the Five Grains] tasted hundreds of grasses, and the medical value of natural resources had been classified and recorded. If the experience and the medical value can be inherited and improved, new findings and innovations will emerge, benefiting human beings.

To end my talk, I would like to share with you a well-known poem called *On the Stork Tower* by Wang Zhihuan (688-742 AD) in the Tang dynasty.

On the Stork Tower[1]

The sun along the mountain bows / The Yellow River seawards flows / You will enjoy a grander sight / By climbing to a greater height.

Let's strive for further improvement to appreciate Chinese culture and find the charm and treasure in TCM!

Finally, I would like to thank all colleagues in China and abroad for their contributions in the discovery, research and clinical application of artemisinin!

Appendix

I am deeply grateful to all my family members for their continuous understanding and support.

I sincerely appreciate your kind attention.

Thank you all!

Chronology of Tu Youyou

1930

Born on December 30, at 508 Kaiming Road, Ningbo city, Zhejiang province

1936-1941   6-11 years old

Entered Chongde private primary school in Ningbo at the age of six

1941   11 years old:

After Ningbo was occupied by the enemy, moved to the Yao residence at 26 Kaiming Road

1941-1943   11-13 years old

Attended Maoxi private primary school in Ningbo

1943-1945   13-15 years old

Went to Qizhen private middle school in Ningbo

1945-1946   15-16 years old

Transferred to the private girls' school, Yongjiang middle school

1948-1950   18-20 years old

Attended Xiaoshi private middle school in Ningbo, where her future husband Li Tingzao was educated from 1944 to 1951

1950-1951   20-21 years old

Attended Ningbo middle school in Zhejiang province

1951-1955   21-25 years old

Admitted to Peking University's school of pharmacy

1955   25 years old

After graduation, was assigned to the Academy of TCM, subordinate to the Ministry of Public Health (now known as the CACMS) in 2005, working in the Institute of Chinese Materia Medica

1959-1962   29-32 years old

Attended the third session of full-time class for doctors of western medicine to learn TCM at the Academy of TCM during her career sabbatical

1963   33 years old

Married Li Tingzao

1965   35 years old

May: Gave birth to her eldest daughter Li Min in Beijing

1968   38 years old

September: Youngest daughter was born in Ningbo

1969   39 years old

21 January: Participated in national cooperative project '523' and then appointed as leader of the research group that undertook the project's research into anti-malaria herbal medicine put forward by the Academy of TCM

April: Completed *Anti-malaria Secret Recipes* containing 640 recipes

July: Worked for the first time in malaria-stricken areas in Hainan

1971   41 years old

October 4: Research group discovered the No. 191 diethyl ether neutral extract sample whose inhibition ratio against plasmodium reached 100%

1972   42 years old

July: Volunteered as 'guinea pig' in clinical test of Artemisia annua extracts

August-December: The research group conducted clinical test of 30 cases of falciparum malaria and vivax malaria in the malaria areas of Changjiang, Hainan province and Beijing 302 Hospital

September 25-November 8: The research group obtained several kinds of crystals through separation

Early December: Mouse malaria experiment found that the crystal obtained on November 8 had obvious effects was called 'artemisia needle-shaped crystal II' at first, but later was called artemisinin

1973   43 years old

March-April: The molecular formula and molecular weight of artemisinin was determined

September-October: Artemisinin was proved to be effective in the first clinical test conducted in the malaria-stricken areas in Changjiang, Hainan province

September: During the production of derivatives of artemisinin, dihydro-artemisinin was found

October: The anti-malaria effects of artemisinin was clinically verified in Hainan

1974   44 years old

January: The institute of Chinese Materia Medica studied artemisinin's molecular structure in cooperation with the Shanghai Institute of Organic Chemistry, and later studied it in cooperation with the institute of Biophysics of the CAS by means of X-ray diffraction

1975   45 years old

November 30: Artemisinin's molecular structure was confirmed

1979   49 years old

Became associate research fellow in the Institute of Chinese Materia Medica of the Academy of TCM

1980   50 years old

Hired as supervisor of postgraduates in the Institute of Chinese Materia Medica of the Academy of TCM at the age of 50

1985   55 years old

Researcher at the Institute of Chinese Materia Medica of the Academy of TCM

1986   56 years old

New drug certificate of artemisinin issued by the Ministry of Health

1992   62 years old

New drug certificate of dihydroartemisinin issued by the Ministry of Health

2001   71 years old

Hired as tutor of doctoral candidates in the Institute of Chinese Materia Medica of the Academy of TCM at the age of 71

2003   73 years old

Received the patent certificate of dihydroartemisinin-containing pharmaceutical composition that cures lupus erythematosus and potosensitive diseases

2004   74 years old

February: Received the patent certificate of dihydroartemisinin, a new anti-malaria drug

June: Obtained the clinical research documents of dihydroartemisinin tablets curing lupus erythematosus

2009   79 years old

Won the third herbal medicine development prize awarded by the Tang Foundation (CACMS)

2011   81 years old

September: Won the Lasker DeBakey clinical medical research award

2015   85 years old

June 15: Won the Warren Albert award granted by the Warren Albert Foundation and Harvard Medical School

October: Won the Nobel prize in physiology or medicine

References

[1] Zhou Xing. Tu Youyou. *The Academic Success Survey of Well-known Chinese Scientists in the 20 Century; Medical Volume; Pharmacy Section*, Science Press, 2013

[2] Tu Youyou. *Sweet Wormwood and Artemisinin-based Drugs*, Chemical Industry Press, 2009

[3] Xu Jizi. *The History of Ningbo*, Zhejiang People's Publishing House, 1986

[4] Li Na. *Tu Youyou and Artemisinin*. Science and Technology Review, 2015, 33 (20)

[5] Jiang Xinjie. *An Overdue Honor for Tu Youyou*, Caixin Weekly, 2011(38)

[6] Li Shanshan. *An Approach to Tu Youyou*, Southern People Weekly, 2011(35)

Afterword

The award of the Nobel prize to Tu Youyou was not only a personal honor but also reflected the vitality of China's science and technology and the great contribution made by TCM to the health of all human beings. This book was published by the People's Publishing House so as to make Tu Youyou's life experience and her good spirit known to the public, such as the persistence in pursuing her dreams, her courage to innovate, selfless contribution, cooperative enterprise and her great endeavors to reach the pinnacle of her career.

CACMS was responsible for editing the book and it was written by many colleagues from *China Women* newspaper, *China Medicine* newspaper and People's Publishing House, among whom Wang Changlu, Wang Manyuan and Chen Tingyi have made great contributions. In order to write the book, we interviewed Tu Youyou and many members of her family, friends and colleagues, and referred to a large amount of materials both at home and aboard. Here, we should express our appreciation to those people and the Institute of Chinese Materia Medica, CACMS for its support. Time being limited, there are still some deficiencies in the book, so we welcome your comments and criticism to improve our work.

Notes

Chapter 4

1. A group of 15 carbon compounds derived by the assembly of three isoprenoid units. They are found mainly in higher plants but also in invertebrates

Appendix

1. Located in Yongji county, Shanxi province

CPSIA information can be obtained
at www.ICGtesting.com
Printed in the USA
BVHW042146160320
575207BV00013B/266